OXFORD MEDICAL PUBLICATIONS

Where's the Evidence?

Controversies in Modern Medicine

Where's the Evidence?

Controversies in Modern Medicine

WILLIAM A. SILVERMAN

Professor of Pediatrics (Retired), Columbia University
Emeritus Member of the Society for Pediatric Research
Emeritus Member of the American Pediatric Society
Emeritus Fellow of the American Academy of Pediatrics
Hon. Founder Fellow of the Royal College of Paediatrics and Child Health

With
a
Foreword
by
David L. Sackett
Professor of Medicine and Director
NHS & R&D Centre for Evidence-Based Medicine, University of Oxford
Consultant in Medicine, John Radcliffe Hospital
Oxford, England, UK

Oxford   New York   Tokyo
OXFORD UNIVERSITY PRESS

Oxford University Press, Great Clarendon Street, Oxford OX2 6DP

Oxford New York
Athens Auckland Bangkok Bogota Bombay
Buenos Aires Calcutta Cape Town Dar es Salaam
Delhi Florence Hong Kong Istanbul Karachi
Kuala Lumpur Madras Madrid Melbourne
Mexico City Nairobi Paris Singapore
Taipei Tokyo Toronto Warsaw
and associated companies in
Berlin Ibadan

Oxford is a trade mark of Oxford University Press

Published in the United States
by Oxford University Press Inc., New York

A catalogue record for this book is available from the British Library

Library of Congress Cataloging in Publication Data
(Data applied for)
ISBN 0 19 262934 4

Typeset by Downdell, Oxford
Printed in Great Britain

To my beloved Roo

*The only one who knows my
bark is worse than my bite.*

*Semper plangere**

* Always complain

FOREWORD

David L. Sackett

Critics can usefully be classified in three ways that guide the readers of their work. First and crudest is by age: young critics are worth at least scanning, for they are likely to bring new ideas and ways of thinking (often laterally), and haven't had enough experience to distort it to back up their prejudices; old critics usually can be ignored, for they often are preoccupied by the need to justify their prior pronouncements (especially when they were wrong).

The second way is by whether the critics take any personal risk in the positions they espouse. When they come from (and especially when they must return to) the front lines where the issues they criticise are played out every day, we can reckon that at least they know what is going on (if not why), and that they are going to have to live with the consequences of both their criticisms and the solutions they propose for them; they deserve thoughtful consideration. When critics are outsiders, especially when they've not even bothered to visit the front lines (my clinical team and patients have welcomed biostatisticians, health economists, a clinical decision analyst, librarians, and policy-makers to our daily rounds and night calls), readers of their criticisms face two additional challenges: at the start, whether they know what they are talking about and, at the end, whether the solutions they propose are even remotely feasible.

The third useful way to classify critics is by their manners, based on Tony Murphy's admonition that criticism, even trenchant criticism, should be an act of purification, not hostility. Critics who have to lose their temper as a prerequisite for taking up their pen, or who cannot devalue an idea or conclusion without having to devalue the person who proposes it, deserve three fates: simply being ignored, being employed for slightly drunken after-dinner light entertainment (I've always preferred a clever conjurer or optimistic tuba player for this purpose), or serving as subjects in studies of the psychopathology of academe. Those who focus on ideas rather than their advocates, and treat those with whom they disagree as worthy individuals who just might be right, deserve our most careful and serious study.

Although Bill Silverman superficially fails the first criterion, he is one of those treasured exceptions to the rule of age. By being true to methods (for determining whether clinical and health care interventions do more good than harm) rather than conclusions (he criticises many of his own), his prior experiences enrich, rather than distort, his criticisms. And he is a role-model for the other two criteria. Immersed for decades in the front lines of neonatal intensive care, he still works with and for the patients who graduated from these awesome, challenging places. And his criticisms, as blunt as any I've encountered, attack ways of thinking and their consequent behaviours, never the worthiness of the clinicians, patients, and policy-makers who think and act in these ways. He even gives space in this book to those who disagree with him and, wonder of wonders, passes up the chance to give the last word!

   I stayed up all night reading this book. Many of you will, too.

Oxford   D.L.S.
September 1997

PREFACE

'How do I know what I think, until I've read what I have written?'

E.M. Forster

In mid-1986, Jean Golding and David Baum were in the throes of a plan to start a new journal, to be published quarterly by Blackwell Scientific, and entitled *Paediatric and Perinatal Epidemiology*. They envisioned a section in this publication, given over to invited commentary, and labelled 'From our own correspondents'. As founding editor, Jean Golding wrote to ask if I would be interested in serving as one these correspondents, with (wondrous!) freedom to write about anything at all; and, she hinted, I might even consider submitting these unedited comments under a *nom de plume*. I replied immediately, and said her offer of a 'soap box' to a chronic complainer like me, was the same as offering free drinks to a drunkard! But I was wary about committing to a regular column; I was reluctant at my age (then 1 year shy of 70) to take on an obligation to write something on schedule rather than on conviction. I promised instead to write occasional pieces, whenever I felt the need to vent my spleen. And this led to the title for these short essays: 'Fumes from the spleen', signed by 'Malcontent'. (I jumped at the chance for masked authorship, because I firmly believed W.H. Auden's remark about writing and writers was doubly relevant in the explication of arguments. An unsigned work, to paraphrase him, forces the reader to respond to the reasoning, not to the reasoner.)

Once I began to write the columns, I quickly found more than enough controversial material to 'fume' about. And I skipped from topic to topic in an attempt to focus on whatever current issue might provoke an argument—in the spirit of what Petr Skrabanek called 'scepticaemia.' (I am grateful to the readers who did write rebuttals [these respondents are listed on p. xvii], and I thank them for now granting permission to include their counter arguments in this book.) Overall, however, I was preoccupied with several recurring themes.

First, I focused on clinicians' resistance to make the distinction between 'observation' and 'experiment'. The importance of paying close attention to the difference, when trying to make sense about the highly variable phenomena that occur at the bedside, goes back to the cautionary advice of Claude Bernard. Awareness of this old problem may, at last, be on the rise. Secondly, I beat the drum to call attention to a relatively recent issue, one that emerged when medicine acquired its immense, first-ever powers to change the expected course of many diseases. Now questions began to turn up about how to wield the unique capabilities wisely. How do we draw a line between 'knowing' (the acquisition of new medical information) and 'doing' (the application of that new knowledge)? What are the long-term consequences (moral, social, economic, and biological) of responding to the demand that we *always* do everything that can be done?

It was painful to see many of the same tragic mistakes in clinical medicine, made over and over again (particularly in the emerging field of neonatology—an area I knew all too well!). I argued repeatedly that errors cannot be avoided when exciting, but untested, new treatments are first introduced, but the number of injured can always be reduced by using the hedging strategy of concurrent controls. The frequent disregard for methodological rigour in clinical studies, I argued, was a sign of our stubborn refusal to recognise that the laws of chance cannot be repealed. (Our dependence on rules imposed by the tenets of probability theory, it has been said, is the same as the need of blind persons for canes: they wouldn't need the aids, if they were able to see ahead!)

Finally, I was preoccupied with the gross maldistribution of power (between patient/family and medical technocrat); the inequality was becoming more disparate than ever. Decisions were, too often, devastating when they were made by those who did not have to live for years with the full consequences of their actions. Signs of increased sensitivity to this problem in recent years have been heartening.

The Introduction, an overview of my main themes, is adapted from the 1994 Windermere Lecture to the British Paediatric Association (reproduced with permission of the BMJ Publishing Group); this is followed by the numbered essays, and I have added afterthoughts to report developments or shifts in views that have taken place since each article was published. The year of original publication is provided in parentheses under each title in the text; the full citation appears at the head of a numbered list under Citations (pp. 204–224), the numbers correspond to superscripts in the text of each essay. The complete references are noted (in alphabetical order) in the Bibliography (pp. 225–247).

I have repeated myself a number of times in the series, and I take refuge in the senior Oliver Wendell Holmes' cheerful, and preemptive, rationalisation. 'What if one does say the same things—of course, in a little different form each time—over and over? If he has anything to say worth saying,' the old man quipped, 'that is just what he ought to do.'

Incredibly, a full 10 years (my entire septuagenarian decade!) have slipped by since I first began to 'fume'. Now I want to acknowledge my debt of gratitude to Jean Golding for providing the platform that allowed me to harangue the readers of *Paediatric and Perinatal Epidemiology* so freely, and for such a protracted period. I am indebted to Rob Schechter who first suggested that the essays be published in book form. I thank Blackwell Science Limited for their generosity in transferring the copyright to Oxford University Press; and I am grateful to Oxford University Press for agreeing that this was the logical time to assemble the 45 essays in book form. The Medical Society of London kindly gave permission to reproduce the Figure (p. 118) taken from a reprint of Richard Asher's Lettsomian Lectures before the society in 1959. Wally Bernstein's sharp eyes saved me from many embarrassing slip-ups, and I am grateful to him. I am obliged to the staff of the Oxford University Press, to Dave Sackett, and to my wife for their suggestions about a title for this book. I want to take this opportunity to thank Dave Sackett on behalf of all clinicians for his inspiring leadership of the evidence-based medicine movement, very personally for his strong letter of support, and for graciously agreeing to write the Foreword to this book. I also want to acknowledge a debt of gratitude to Iain Chalmers for his friendship over the years and for providing unfailing inspiration. My close friend Mac Holliday debated with me (and provided much needed moral support) on the innumerable and wonderful hiking trails in Point Reyes over the entire decade during which these essays were written—I am very grateful to him.

I want to tell my wife (in a separate paragraph on this very public page) how grateful I am for her editorial wizardry, how much I have treasured our 52 years together, and how much I love her. Thanks for everything, Roo!

Jan 1998   W.A.S.
California

Contents

Abbreviations

AIDS acquired immunodeficiency syndrome
AMA American Medical Association
AZT zidovudine
CAST Cardiac Arrhythmia Suppression Study
CONSORT Consolidated Standards of Reporting Trials
CPP Collaborative Perinatal Project (US)
CPR cardiopulmonary resuscitation
CNS central nervous system
DES diethylstilbestrol
EBM evidence-based medicine
ECMO extracorporeal membrane oxygenation
FDA Food and Drug Administration (US)
ICU intensive care unit (adult)
IOM Institute of Medicine (US)
IRB institutional review board
LBW low birthweight
MEDLINE National Library of Medicine Database (US)
MORI polling organisation (UK)
NICU neonatal intensive care unit
NIH National Institutes of Health (US)
POW prisoner of war
RCT randomised clinical trial
RDS respiratory distress syndrome
ROP retinopathy of prematurity
SUPPORT Study to Understand Prognosis and Preferences for
  Outcomes and Risks of Treatment
UK United Kingdom
US United States

Respondents

William E. Benitz, Associate Professor of Pediatrics, Clinical Director of Neonatal Intensive Care Unit. Lucile Packard Children's Hospital at Stanford University School of Medicine, Palo Alto, California, USA.

Peter W. Fowlie, Consultant Paediatrician, Ninewells Hospital and Medical School, University of Dundee, Dundee, UK.

Amnon Goldworth, Senior Medical Ethicist, Lucile Packard Children's Hospital, Stanford University School of Medicine, Palo Alto, California, USA.

John D. Lantos, Associate Professor of Pediatrics and Medicine, Associate Director, MacLean Center for Clinical Medical Ethics, University of Chicago Pritzker School of Medicine, Chicago, Illinois, USA.

Saroj Saigal, Professor, Department of Pediatrics, McMaster University, Hamilton, Ontario, Canada.

John C. Sinclair, Professor, Departments of Pediatrics and of Clinical Epidemiology and Biostatistics, McMaster University, Hamilton, Ontario, Canada.

John L. Watts, Professor, Department of Pediatrics, McMaster University, Hamilton, Ontario, Canada.

William B. Weil, Jr., Professor (Emeritus), Department of Pediatrics and Human Development, Michigan State University College of Human Medicine, East Lansing, Michigan, USA.

Introduction: medicine's dilemma at the end of the twentieth century

Science teaches us to doubt and, in ignorance, to refrain.

Claude Bernard

'Do something, *anything!*' is a universal cry for help at the onset of pain and suffering of illness. Throughout all of human history, 'healers' have responded with imagination and boundless enthusiasm.

I first saw an instructive example of this 'therapeutic imperative' in New York City during a poliomyelitis epidemic in the late summer of 1944—more than 50 years ago. I was a resident at The Babies Hospital of Columbia University when the outbreak occurred. It quickly became the largest epidemic in the city's history; and an entire floor of the hospital was set aside for polio patients. In a back ward, we had four cumbersome Drinker respirators (the so-called 'iron-lung' machines), and they were fully occupied for almost six weeks by a succession of patients with bulbar involvement, the highly lethal form of the disease.

The weather that summer was brutally hot and humid. In those days, hospitals were not air-conditioned: the wards were like steam baths. Ambient conditions on the polio ward were made even more uncomfortable by huge copper vats of water, boiling day and night to keep the Kenny packs steaming hot. These packs, made of woollen cloth, were wrapped around the affected limbs of patients according to a regimen set-out by Sister Kenny, an Australian nurse. The continuous applications of hot, moist packs were meant to relieve the immediate pain of muscular spasm; and, more importantly, it was believed they would reduce the amount of residual paralysis.

On the night I remember best, during that harrowing summer, the ward nurses, wearing masks and floor-length isolation gowns reminded me of a painting of Florence Nightingale's dedicated angels of mercy on a hospital ward during the Crimean War. They seemed to be suspended a few inches above the floor in the darkened wards, as they glided silently in a continuous shuttle between the steaming cauldrons and the naked patients lying in the ward beds. A little after midnight, two patients, in respirators, died in quick succession. We were physically and emotionally exhausted.

About 3 a.m., to our amazement, the attending consultant arrived on the floor, and asked to be taken on a complete ward round. He was very drunk. His gait was unsteady and his necktie, knotted perfectly, was turned 180 degrees and hung down the back of his shirt. But he was quite sedate, his speech was not slurred, and he was completely lucid. After we reported the details of the two deaths, we walked from bed to bed with flashlights, and he made whispered comments about each patient. He kept to a consistent theme: over and over again, he pointed out the extreme variation in the extent of paralysis among the affected children. Treatment with Kenny packs did seem to relieve the pain, he conceded, but it was impossible to know if, or indeed, how much decrease in paralysis could be attributed to treatment in this notoriously unpredictable disorder. It was well known, he reminded us, that more than half of young children with acute poliomyelitis were left with no residual motor deficit. Given the extreme variability, he asked, 'How could we ever hope to recognise a small *increase* in paralysis among the Kenny-pack-treated children?'

As I look back, a half-century ago, to this bizarre, middle-of-the-night ward round led by my drunken, but very canny teacher, I recognise this as a peak experience in my medical education. But it did take years to realise that his question about the safety, as well as the efficacy of Kenny-pack treatment made a crucially-important point: Therapy must always be seen as a sword with at least two edges. His concern for the well-being of our patients was much more responsible than our emotional preoccupation, which was driven by the fear of not doing *enough*! 'How can we, in good conscience, withhold packs from half of our patients,' we thought to ourselves, 'if there is even the slightest hope for improvement in outlook?' It was this last fear-filled question that stood in the way of finding out whether Kenny packs were helping or, in fact, harming our patients. At the time, I was indignant. How could this drunken sceptic be so cruel as to question our heroic efforts to help these children? No other treatment was available! I thought it was malicious to point out the remote possibility that a measure so simple and so-seemingly benign as the hot packs might worsen outlook. The nurses and the families were completely convinced the packs were work-ing miracles: all improvement was the result of the Kenny treatment, all failures were explained away by the claim that treatment was not started soon enough.

During this very same period, it was this uncritical faith in another untested treatment that was responsible for the 12-year delay in recognis-ing the horrendous result of an apparently simple act: turning up the flow of oxygen—a long-trusted, life-giving gas—into the incubators for prematurely-born infants. Only after the oxygen/blindness disaster,[1] did we recognise that the soft-headed reasoning about cause-and-effect in medicine had changed very little over a period of two-millennia.

In ancient Rome, Galen made a sweeping claim about his infallible treatment; it had a familiar ring. He said,

> All who drink of this treatment recover in a short time,
> Except those whom it does not help, who all die.
> It is obvious, therefore, that it fails only in incurable cases.

Soon after the polio experience, the powerful antibiotic drugs and the corticosteroids arrived on the scene: they ushered in an unprecedented period of optimism. As I take a long look back at this era, I think it demonstrated what might be called 'The Opiate Effect of Success.' The parade of spectacular results, after use of the new miracle drugs, led to a Galen-like dogmatic slumber. Success after success led to a weakening of a spirit of doubt of the kind my tipsy consultant tried so hard to encourage on that bizarre night on the polio ward.

The slam-bang effects of the new agents in the first decade or two after World War II, led to an exuberant 'let's-try-it-and-see' attitude. At every opportunity, I have spoken and written about the unbridled therapeutic sprees and unexpected treatment disasters during this uncritical period, particularly the debacles involving highly vulnerable prematurely-born neonates. I will resist the compulsion to recite the gloomy story again, and mention only how very dangerous it is to use treatments widely before they are subjected to rigorous comparative tests.

The lessons have, for the most part, been learned. There is no question that the explosive increase in medical knowledge in the past several decades has led to the development of safe, and increasingly effective interventions. The expected time-course and outcome of a growing number of human afflictions can be modified, as never before in the history of our species.

There is a rumbling note of uneasiness that underlies present-day medical progress: the more we know in medicine, the more questions we encounter about what to do with the hard-won information. One critic has pointed out[1] that 'medicine has entered a new stage of its history; one where the successes, and not the failures, are the main source of our problems.' And these 'failures of success' are seen, in caricature, at both extremes of the life span.

I can recall an early victory in the 1960s,[2] when neonatal intensive care was just getting organised in the US. A dedicated team of nurses and paediatricians (they were not yet called neonatologists) was successful in 'saving' an 800 gram infant who developed one life-threatening complication after another. Three months and several tens-of-thousands of dollars after birth, the baby was sent home to a cold-water flat in a run-down section of the city. Within a week, we heard that the infant died when a rat chewed off its nose.

Looking back at our well-intentioned, never-say-die fight to keep this marginally-viable infant alive, I cannot in good conscience, label the struggle as an act of pure benevolence. I am forced to ask, 'Was our benevolence simply a form of self-gratification? Did we have a genuine impulse to do good, or merely a compulsion to feel good?'

One of the nurses in the special care unit described the situation faced by all young caretakers with a 'rescue fantasy.' She said, 'When I come home, dead tired, after working very hard to keep these small infants alive, I have a hard time falling asleep; I keep asking myself, "Am I doing it for the baby, or am I doing it for myself?"'

A small group of humanists met a few years ago to discuss some general questions about social policy.[3] They soon found themselves talking about a society's responsibility for the care of its dependants. They quickly recognised that a virtuous claim to be acting benevolently in these situations was becoming increasingly suspect. 'If the last refuge of the scoundrel was once patriotism,' an observer noted, 'now it appeared to be the activity of "doing good" for others. . .' (that is to say, acting in what he/she *defines* as the best interest of someone else).

The value of the paternalistic model in social work and in medicine needs to be questioned. 'Where,' it was asked, 'should the authority of the care-giver leave off, and the rights of the cared-for begin?' For better or worse, it was observed, 'social thought and social policy in our society seems to be in the process of making a startling break with some very old and hallowed ideas.'

A judge, who heard that the topic of 'benevolence' had been discussed at the conference, criticised the group for even considering that the idea 'was anything more than the exercise of power in disguise.' The criticism forces us to re-examine some long-accepted notions about the proper limits of medicine's domain. For example, in the field I know best, we need to determine the extent to which neonatal intensive care is directly responsive to problems brought to the experts by families. Are these highly-skilled specialists responding to needs, or are they creating needs to which they respond? We need to know, I suggest, whether neonatal medicine's enormous increase in technical power has allowed it to become coercive.

It is a mistake to suppose that any technical innovation has one, and only one, effect. 'Every technical development is both a blessing and a burden,' said one social critic:[4] 'not either-or, but this-and-that.' As Thoreau once observed, 'We need to ask whether our inventions are but improved means to an unimproved end.'

During his tenure as Minister of Health in Greece, Spyros Doxiadis recognised that many ethical dilemmas turn up in present-day health promotion. Before his death, he wrote movingly about the need to explore such conflicts.[5]

The problem of deciding how to mount organised efforts to reduce mortality and morbidity in socially disadvantaged, high-risk human populations, I would like to call it 'The Doxiadis Dilemma, brings me to the *fin de siècle* questions: How do we go about drawing a line between 'knowing' and 'doing' in medicine at the end of the twentieth century? When do we know enough about the full medical and social consequences of our interventions to proceed with confidence?

In the US, a stark example of the dilemma is seen in the contrast between the enormous amount of effort and resources deployed to provide unlimited intensive treatment for marginally-viable neonates, and the piddling amounts of social support and money made available to improve the living conditions of overwhelmed families who must care for the fragile survivors. In too many instances, the pregnancies were not planned, the children were not wanted, and a disproportionate number of the distressed families are socially disadvantaged. A disturbing number of prematurely-born infants are born to the poor, to the unemployed, to welfare recipients, to under-educated school leavers, to the medically under-served, to teen-age mothers (themselves frequently unloved children in dysfunctional families). The brittle families are poorly fed, and inadequately housed in the midst of drug-ridden, violent neighbourhoods. The stress of daily survival is endlessly corrosive.

Unlike the past, when rescue efforts were ineffective, and the parents' wishes to withhold even simple supportive care for a marginally-viable infant were almost always respected, the present situation is unprecedented in all of human history. With the sharp increase in medical knowledge and in development of highly effective interventions, there has been a remarkable shift in attitude and in medical action. The results have been dramatic, as measured by the survival of infants who were abandoned only a short time ago as 'pre-viable' or 'hopelessly malformed.'

The full social costs of this extremely expensive, aggressive, high-tech war on neonatal mortality have, for the most part, not been measured. The situation reminds me of the bitter lyrics of an old anti-war song,[6]

Once the rockets are up, who cares where they come down?
'That's not my department,' says Wernher von Braun.

A growing number of voices are asking about the effects on families and on the community at large. They question the advisability of making intense technical efforts to prolong the lives of all infants with complete disregard of the far-reaching social consequences. The myopic outlook of never-say-die neonatal warfare reminds me of the attitudes in the disastrous war in Vietnam. One of our officers justified the torching of all straw huts in a settlement with the explanation, 'We had to destroy the village to save it.'

The decisions about how far we can, or must, go in the deployment of high-powered medical weaponry—the line between 'knowing' and 'doing' in medicine—should not, in my opinion, be made by specialists. Medical warfare is not all that different from conventional war ('the continuation of politics by other means'[7]); it is much too important to be left to the experts.

Freidson examined the limits of professional knowledge from a sociologist's point of view.[8] He concluded that when decisions are essentially 'moral or evaluative, rather than substantive, layman have as much, if not more to contribute than experts.' This assumption, he argued, 'reflects the property of equality in a free society: equality, not of ability, not of knowledge, nor of means; but that of moral equality.' A legal scholar recently came to a similar conclusion.[9]

As we approach the twenty-first century, on the threshold of the genetics revolution, the increasing technical power of modern medicine is, I suggest, on a collision course with an equally significant revolution in the composition of modern societies brought on by massive migrations. Societies are becoming explicitly and stridently pluralistic.

Medicine's monolithic view of what constitutes a good life clashes, inevitably, with the innumerable and kaleidoscopic views of the multi-ethnic populations in many countries of the Western world. A bioethicist has pointed out[10] that medicine has emerged as a secular profession treating individuals drawn from many cultural and religious backgrounds. As a result, he argued, it must adopt a neutral stance as it attempts to respond to the expressed needs of a wide variety of religious believers and non-believers; whites, blacks, browns and yellows; homosexuals and heterosexuals; the able and the disabled...; the numbers of sub-categories that are proclaiming the right of self-determination are growing. In choosing among different possible modes of medical treatment, or in rejecting all specific treatment, the cultural subgroups, families and individuals are demanding the right to choose their own sickness styles and their own death styles; to write, in essence, their own life stories.[11]

The collision between medicine and the emerging heterogeneous societies need not be a disastrous encounter. In fact, I see this as an opportunity for a newly-powerful medicine to step back and examine itself: Where are we going?

We must be aware of the need for restraint; and our capacity for restraint must be proportional to the power we now command. Questions about interventions often begin with, How should we proceed?, rather than, Why are we doing this? What are medicine's goals? Is medicine's primary aim to increase the length of life? Or is it to reduce the amount of pain and suffering? And who is empowered to choose when these ends are mutually exclusive?

For clues to some answers, I suggest, we need to turn back to a time when doctors were among the persons most revered in communties. The much admired objectives of the medical profession in that halcyon age, are spelled out in very few words at the base of a statue at Saranac Lake, New York, honouring Edward Trudeau (1848–1915) for his devoted care of patients with tuberculosis before the antibiotic era:

To cure sometimes; to help often; to console always.

1

Selective ethics
(1987)

> ... our path is cumbered with guesses, presumptions and conjectures, the untimely and sterile fruitage of minds which cannot bear to wait for the facts, and are ready to forget that the use of hypothesis lies not in the display of ingenuity but in the labour of verification.'
>
> Sir Clifford Allbutt

Smithells' lament voiced over a decade ago[1] ('I need permission to give a new drug to half my patients, but not to give it to them all.') points to a situation that is akin to Alice's observation concerning one of her puzzling adventures in Wonderland: It grows 'curiouser and curiouser' by the year.

Now comes a report about medical research with children[2] that takes notice of innovative therapy ('performance of a new or non-standard intervention as all or part of a therapeutic activity and not as part of a formal research project'). And, the report advises, there should be a limit on the number of times such interventions are used on children, before they are submitted as formal research projects to ethics committees. Commendable advice, but why, one wonders, did the Institute of Medical Ethics Working Group stop short of a call for mandatory pre-review of the initial explorations? It clearly labels the pilot efforts as 'haphazard', and it is well known that this is a grey area of clinical activity. When first results of exploration seem to be favourable (as compared with past experience) the innovation is quickly baptised as 'standard practice.' Years may go by before the claim is put to the test and, as happens much too often, the exciting treatment is found to be useless or harmful.

Innovators in the growing field of neonatal medicine seem to be particularly unbridled. Results of their bold preliminary efforts are accepted eagerly by prestigious medical journals and reported breathlessly in news media. The slow boring job of formal evaluation using concurrent controls, is left to others. (The situation is reminiscent of the scene in Thornton Wilder's 'The Skin of Our Teeth,'[3] a tongue-in-cheek allegorical play about the history of humankind in which the 'Everyman' character, a Mr. George Antrobus, announces, 'Three cheers, I have invented the wheel.' When his wife asks, 'A wheel? What's a wheel?', he replies, 'Any booby can figure that out, but I thought of it first.')

Why, for example, are neonates chosen to receive the hoped-for benefits of an untried treatment during the period of initial 'haphazard' exploration, not provided with the same safeguards recommended for others? Enrolees in authentic trials, it cannot be emphasised enough, are protected by formal prior-reviews. And, even more curious, why does there appear to be so little concern for babies treated outside the context of a not-yet-completed parallel-treatment trial? These exercises are undertaken because risks and benefits of the innovation have not yet been established.

There is little hope that the schizophrenic situation in neonatal medicine will change until there is a change in the 'gung ho!' attitude in this fast moving field. Although neonatologists are not unique, their outlook is particularly intense because of what they see as an urgent need to save lives and to prevent life-long handicap. There is impatience with the delays resulting from demands of methodologists. These formalists insist that new proposals pass tough tests before they are released for use in the desperately sick babies not enrolled in controlled clinical exercises.

Resistance to the dictum that every new treatment must be subjected to the discipline of a true experiment seems to be related to a widely-held belief that 'the formality is required only to convince others of what we, the innovators, *know* from careful and systematic observation to be true.' Unfortunately, the oft-made argument against critical tests fails to mention that the experimental format is the only way we have of protecting babies from what is *not known* about innovations. Uncertainty is inescapable—vagaries are encountered at every turn in medical study and, authoritative opinion to the contrary notwithstanding, there are no criteria that allow us to judge when we know everything about clinical phenomena.

After three years studying the conduct of present-day medical research with children, the Working Group of the Institute of Medical Ethics concluded that planned studies are both desirable and necessary to promote health and well being, and recommendations were made to ensure that youngsters enrolled in research projects are adequately protected against unreasonable risks. The project deserves the highest praise; and yet one cannot help wishing that the review of potential risks for relatively small numbers of participants in planned projects had been extended. What is needed is an examination of hazards endured by the very large numbers of children—neonates are, once more, a good example—who receive treatments every day that have never been subjected to rigorous evaluation. Recurrent therapeutic disasters in the modern era provide convincing testimony about the risks of accepted, but unevaluated, practices. Unexpected hazards are often uncovered late, and they are by no means inconsequential.

Perhaps in further reviews of ethical issues surrounding research activities involving children, consideration will be given to the proposition that consequences of medical error in a very young child are likely to be more serious than in adults; and that repercussions are felt for a larger proportion of total life time. If the premise is true, it surely follows that there is an ethical imperative here: We must insist on the highest standards of evidence in studies involving the youngest human beings; and, since there is no short route to this goal, we must be prepared to be patient. Moreover, if the current headlong rush to the perfection of means is slowed, perhaps there will be time for critical examination of the confusion of goals in neonatal medicine where activities have become dangerously fanatical. (Fanaticism, Santayana once noted, consists of redoubling your efforts after forgetting your aims.)

(1997)

Since the above complaint was written a decade ago, uncontrolled explorations of new treatments in neonates have not been curbed appreciably. For example, the large multicenter trial of Cryotherapy for Retinopathy of Prematurity (CRYO-ROP) demonstrated the effectiveness of this intervention in suppressing the retinopathy, and in hastening its involution. But even before the long-term results of CRYO-ROP were reported,[1] a new approach—laser photocoagulation—was introduced. This new unevaluated technique was quickly accepted as 'standard therapy,' because the method was technically easier to apply than the cryoprobe, particularly in the smallest babies requiring treatment that may extend close to the macula. Moreover, unlike the conservative criteria for treatment in the CRYO-ROP trial, many more mild instances of ROP are now being treated with laser photocoagulation. As a result, many vascular changes in the retina that would be expected to resolve completely and spontaneously, are now treated by ablation.

Despite concerns about the risk of cataracts as a complication of laser treatment (and knowledge that, unlike adults, cataract surgery in a neonate may have catastrophic consequences on visual development),[2] no attempts have been made to compare the relative risks of cryotherapy vs laser coagulation in a concurrent randomised trial. It is hard to deny that Sir Clifford Allbutt's call for the 'labour of verification' continues to go unheeded.

2
Does a difference make a difference?
(1987)

'The most important maxim for data analysis, and one which statisticians have shunned, is this: Far better an approximate answer to the right question, which is often vague, than an exact answer to the wrong question, which can always be made precise.

John W. Tukey[1]

More than eighty years ago, Bernard Shaw wrote (with pen dipped in vitriol) that the doctor of his day drew 'disastrous conclusions from his clinical experience because he has no conception of scientific method, and believes, like any rustic, that the handling of evidence needs no expertness.'[2] Cynics will say that, except for the awareness of male bias in the use of gender pronouns, nothing has changed. But fair witnesses can point to clear signs that the doctor of today is developing a deep respect for the formalities used in the evaluation of everyday experience. Indeed, it can be argued that the medical profession has been cowed into unhealthy submission by the confidence and calculus of number jugglers (especially the emphasis on hypothesis-testing rather than estimation of the size-of-difference of a measured outcome between groups),[3] and by the flaunting of P values to impart an aura of mathematical proof.[4]

Conscientious physicians seeking fair appraisals of treatment possibilities tumbling out of today's cornucopia of proposals need to keep their feet planted in the real world. At the end of the day, patients, their immediate surrogates, their families and the community at large need to be convinced that all of the heady medical activity is in the sufferer's best interest. The need for realism is seen very clearly in the effect-size problem in the design of clinical trials of compared treatments: What *is* an important difference in outcomes?

When planning the dimensions of a clinical trial, researchers are required (in the Neyman–Pearson 'game'[5]) to provide a precise answer to the value-laden question: 'What is the smallest difference between treatments you think is important enough to find?' And they must wrestle with two uncomfortable questions about levels of error protection: (i) If you say, at the end of a trial, 'There is an important difference in outcomes,' how large a risk of being wrong are you willing to take? and (ii) How large a risk are you willing to take in missing the actual existence of an important difference by declaring, 'There is no statistically significant difference'? It is hard to escape the uneasy feeling that the underlying motive of the need for caution on the part of the investigator, when he/she replies to the posed question, has more to do with self-protection (the researcher's reputation is at stake) than with the need to consider overall social consequences.

'Methods' sections in reports of clinical trials rarely provide the prior arguments used: i) when the decision was made to define the smallest difference thought to be important; and ii) how the decision was made to accept stated levels of uncertainty about conclusions. Silence about the details fuels suspicion that the agreements are often narrowly defined. Many investigators give the impression they are embattled. As noted earlier, they seem to think they are forced to conduct formal trials *only* to persuade sceptical rivals that the new treatment 'works.' The beleaguered view was revealed several years ago in a rare confession, 'We're convinced that treatment A is far better than B, but we can't convince Doctors X, Y and Z unless we have a randomised clinical study.'[6]

Where is the public choice in the matter of what shall be considered an important difference in treatment outcomes? Surely the preferences of those whose lives and well-being are directly affected need to be taken into account if a treatment of medical interest is to be transformed into something of social value. Is it not time to insist that there be public involvement in formulating the exact criteria to decide that 'treatment A is far better than B?' Approaches used to quantitate the degree of preference for health states (e.g. adaptations of the standard gamble technique for measuring preferences[7]) provide a model for incorporating community views in clinical trials design. The additional planning time required to obtain public consultation will be well worth the investment if questions asked in treatment trials begin to approach the one proposed by John Burroughs for evaluating the outcome of all human interventions:[8] 'Is life sweeter? That is the test.'

(1997)

The question of how to improve on Burrough's subjective test of 'an important difference' in treatment outcomes still goes answered. The failure would not have surprised the American Chief Justice, Oliver

Wendell Holmes: 'Most people think dramatically,' he once observed, 'not quantitatively.'

What needs to be overcome is a naive 'all-*and*-none concept'; the unrealistic expectation that an effective treatment will cure virtually all patients with a specified illness; and, conversely, practically none of the patients with this illness will improve without specific treatment. But help is on the way. It is encouraging to see that in the past few years, the advocates of evidence-based medicine at McMaster University and at Oxford University have been examining the effect-size question in considerable detail.[1] They have been devising ways to express quantitative estimates of effectiveness that focus on *the limitations* of treatments. The aim is to make this realistic information available to practitioners, patients, families, communities, and even to new players on the medical scene, the bureaucrats in managed care. (Increasingly and ominously, the latter administrators are making many crucial decisions about treatments.)

One innovative approach, introduced by the Canadians, is the '*number needed to treat*' concept.[2] They cite, as an example, a parallel-treatment trial of hypertension in which 20% of enrolled patients allotted to the placebo group suffered a cerebral stroke within a five-year interval of observation; the risk of this adverse event was reduced to 12% among patients with moderate hypertension who received active treatment. The estimate of the absolute risk reduction in the trial was $0.20 - 0.12 = 0.08$; and the reciprocal of this number, $1.0 / 0.08 = 13$, provides an estimate of the number needed to treat (NNT). The practitioner uses this sober information about limits to tell decision makers that for patients with moderate hypertension, one would need to treat about 13 patients for five years with the expectation of preventing one stroke. On the other hand, from the results in patients with mild hypertension, the risk of stroke was reduced from a baseline of 0.015 in the placebo-treated group, to 0.009 in patients who received specific treatment. Here, the magnitude of limitation is unmistakable: to prevent one stroke the estimate of NNT is 167.

This easy-to-grasp information (and additional quantitative statements: confidence intervals of NNT, to indicate the imprecision of the study sample; and threshold NNT, to take into account the level of impact that warrants a recommendation for treatment) should help to inform the decisions made by all concerned about the treatment of patients with disorders that vary widely in different practice settings and from patient to patient.

3

Prescription for disaster
(1988)

Rational systems extended to the extremes of their rationality
often turn into nightmares.

Jorge Luis Borges

In recent years, accomplishments in the burgeoning field of perinatal
medicine have been dramatic—some would say near-miraculous. For
concrete evidence to support the expansive claims, one need only point
to the striking increase in survival of infants who were abandoned only
a short time ago as 'pre-viable' or 'hopelessly malformed.'

The abrupt shift in attitude, in action, and in conviction of professional
caretakers is remarkable. But, we must ask, does the community at large
share the rescue fantasy of the hard-working teams who undertake the
new never-say-die efforts? Do those most directly affected, the parents
who must live with the long-term consequences of present-day heroics,
share the neonatologists' enthusiasm for the unprecedented increase in
survival rates for the smallest and the most malformed neonates?

The questions remind us that medicine, like the Roman god Janus, has a
dual countenance. One face is preoccupied with the question, How do we
make sense out of information? We have more than 350 years' experience
with an effective approach to this problem—Galileo called it *il cimento*,
the ordeal. All knowledge claims are subjected to the ordeal of relentless
criticism by sceptical co-workers. If a claim remains standing after all of
the abuse, it is adopted as a temporary, but often quite useful 'working
truth.' The strength of the claim is measured by the number and the force
of attempts to dislodge it.

The second face of medicine looks at the question, How do we transform new medical information into something of social value? Here
we have little experience because, until recently, interventions were so
ineffective, the question was moot. There is growing awareness that a
claim in this sphere must also run the gauntlet; but there is a crucial
difference. Here, withering criticism of a claim about the utility of a
medical action *must* come from sceptics in the community, if we are to

distinguish between a half-way technical solution and a solid claim of improvement in general welfare. What needs to be recognised is the need for a critical review of neonatal medicine's growing power of social control. Bates reminds us[1] that no extensive and continuing communication has taken place between the new specialists and the rest of society. In effect, intensive care of the smallest and most seriously malformed neonates is unreviewed and unlegislated social policy.

A flood of news items, television programmes, magazine articles, and a number of books have subjected intensive neonatal care as practised in the US to searing criticism. Parents,[2] journalists,[3,4] sociologists,[5] and political scientists[6] have described some incredible situations that have turned up in special care baby units in that country. (The horror stories remind us of the need to remember the admonition of Thomas Jefferson: 'When the state of the patient goes beyond the real limits of [the physician's] art, his office is to be a watchful, but quiet spectator of the operations of nature.')

One news report[7] about an infant born 17 weeks before term and weighing 482 grams at birth, quoted one of the baby's many doctors as follows:

> ... she has been plagued with frequent kidney failures, liver problems that defy textbook definition, and the usual lung problems ... at seven months after delivery she is hanging in there. We have kept the umbilical artery catheter in her aorta all the way, so her hyperalimentation has been intra-arterial ... she can't suck because of the endotracheal tube ... of course, she has been constantly on PEEP [positive end-expiratory pressure] ... But with no spontaneous breathing, all mechanical ventilation, her lungs are pretty damaged now.

What did her parents think, what are we all to think, about this impressive flexing of life-prolonging hardware?

'Rescuers' define their all-out efforts with narrowly interpreted legal and theological arguments—even when their whole-hearted dedication is not matched by an equal commitment on the part of the parents and the community. What are the long-term consequences of inequalities in commitment?

One survey of infants leaving a special care baby unit indicated that such graduates are at relatively high risk for neglect, abuse and death in the post-neonatal period.[8] There is a strong suspicion that this dismal state of affairs is due, in no small part, to what has been called a 'continuum of caretaking casualty.'[9] Parents with marginal financial and emotional resources are often overwhelmed by the survival of a sickly or malformed baby—the situation becomes a prescription for disaster.

The concept that all 'expected losses' of human pregnancies should be prevented is a completely new idea in the long history of the human species. The chronicle of efforts to accomplish the new social goal has been marked by continuous conflict: The attitudes of parents have not always agreed with authorities. On the whole, parents have acted on the assumption that each baby is a personal possession. They are the ones, they argue, to decide whether to invest the economic and emotional resources needed to transform their completely dependent biological creation into an independent social being. The power struggle over the issue of autonomy is heightened at the birth of a seriously compromised infant.

Students of human behaviour hold out little hope that solutions will last if they are imposed on parents. When ideal solutions are sought on issues for which there is no humane solution, Peter Marris observed,[10] outcomes are often 'widely destructive.'

(1997)

The first book-length account of parents' criticism of neonatal intensive care described what they termed 'the long dying' of their marginally-viable infant born in 1976.[1] Nineteen years later, a mother has written about a similar experience; and her recent book indicates that scepticism and controversy continue to hound these neonatal dramas.[2] 'Family members are not the only ones traumatized,' she writes. 'Even when allowing a baby to die is the most humane and medically appropriate alternative to keeping her alive, doctors, out of fear of legal retribution or social castigation, will choose to prolong life. This dilemma of conscience was experienced by [our child's] doctors; and our wish to have all treatment withdrawn ... was thwarted by their dilemma. Everyone's dilemma.'

Unhappily, the uncertainties are even more tangled than recognised by the parent-critics. For example, a variation in mortality (in a survey of 62 American neonatal intensive care units, reported in 1997[3]) suggested to the investigators that 'the effectiveness of medical care varies among units.' But the finding may also reflect a disparity in decision-making at critical moments in the rescue of the most fragile neonates. Simple fairness demands that parents must be told about the extent of any difference in attitudes and actions of the intensivists who are shaping the young family's future so indelibly.

4

Therapeutic mystique (1988)

Fill your mouth with milk and shake it until it becomes butter, in this way at least three out of four toothaches cease immediately and without fail.

Eighteenth century remedy[1]

Few would deny that to a greater or lesser extent there is an element of suggestion in the therapeutic process. Although evidence on the point is largely anecdotal, a placebo effect probably does play a role in all treatments.[2-5] Patients appear to respond best when they 'have faith' in their doctors. Doctors, in turn, seem to be more effective when they 'believe' in the treatments they prescribe. Richard Asher once noted that a doctor's self-confidence is an invaluable part of the therapeutic relationship: 'If you are certain you are right and if you can convince the patient that you are right, then whether you really are right or not often makes very little difference.'[6] In some instances, the effectiveness of a new drug depends *entirely* on a doctor's confident expectations.[7] Frequently there is mutual reinforcement: Patients have a remarkably intuitive ability to sense what is wanted of them and they provide it.

The therapeutic mystique creates an ethical dilemma when a new treatment is proposed to replace the trusted standard. It is a necessary condition for participation in a planned trial of parallel treatments, the bioethicists assert, that clinical investigators be in a state of genuine uncertainty regarding the relative merits of the old versus the newly-proposed intervention (this balanced doubt has been dubbed 'equipoise'[8]). When a doctor believes that patients in one arm of a planned trial are to be provided with better treatment, he is, seemingly, disqualified from participation. Under conventional rules, he cannot, in good faith, represent to patients that treatment choices in the trial are equal.[9]

There *is* an irresolvable conflict between the ethical requirement that a patient must always be offered the best treatment known, and the equivocal choice on-offer in a planned trial.[10] The formal exercise is carried out in the hope that the newly-proposed treatment will surpass the accepted regimen.

Freedman has come up with a suggestion that may help to resolve the knotty problem. He proposes that the time has come to question the high moral status accorded an individual doctor's treatment preference—particularly when that choice is backed by weak evidence (e.g. uncontrolled experience, untested extrapolations from pre-clinical studies, a 'gut feeling', and so on). Personal and idiosyncratic decisions about 'best treatment known' cannot be defended, Freedman correctly asserts, when there is an honest disagreement among experts about the relative benefit of treatment alternatives. The ethics of medical practise grant no moral standing to a treatment preference, no matter how staunchly held, when that opinion is based on anything less than evidence publicly presented and convincing to the community of doctors. Good medicine is defined by professional consensus.

It follows from these arguments that a doctor with a decided treatment preference may, in good conscience, participate in a controlled clinical trial when he/she acknowledges that there is insufficient evidence to judge 'best action' and when that state of doubt is disclosed to the patient.

The acceptance of uncertainty undermines a comforting relationship between doctors and their patients—confidence in the physician's capability has served well throughout medical history. For thousands of years, doctors were held in high esteem and were sought after by those in the highest places in social hierarchies. Doctors were credited with cures, but we know now they were prescribing drugs and procedures that were completely ineffective or dangerous. The curious paradox makes sense if we acknowledge that physicians were themselves effective therapeutic agents.[11] Houston commented that it was the skill of physicians in dealing with the emotions of their patients (the much vaunted 'art of medicine') which sustained the medical profession throughout the centuries.[12] The 'art' was impressive—patients were willing to pay for perceived relief and cures. It was the faith of both doctor and patient in the medication or medical action that seemed to provide hoped-for improvement.

Needless to say, doctors feel threatened when they are asked to abandon the time-honoured essence of their 'art'. A doctor's confession of uncertainty seems to violate an unwritten declaration: 'Trust me!'[13] Indeed, such 'optimistic biases,' Parson suggests,[14] are very general and fundamental in human social organisation. The mental set is probably responsible for the compelling belief in the efficacy of interventions, and magical beliefs and practises in many situations associated with uncertainty. There are, in these circumstances, very strong emotional interests in the utility of action. Concern about giving up therapeutic methods, abilities or beliefs that are perceived as successful may be the greatest single obstacle to doctors participating in clinical trials.[15]

The dilemma comes at an unprecedented time in medical history. For the first time doctors are armed with a wide array of highly effective interventions.[16] In the past they were virtually unarmed but highly respected. Now faith in these unquestionably effective healers seems to be fading. How strange!

(1997)

The conflict between the convictions of individual practitioners and the doubts of methodologists is often intense, particularly when evaluating surgical treatment. A recent cautionary example involves the prevailing opinions of urologists in different countries, concerning the quality of evidence in support of radical excision for early cancer of the prostate.

Swedish urologists recently reported[1] prospective observations on 'the natural history of initially-untreated prostate cancer' in a population-based cohort of afflicted men with the early stages of the disease. Among 223 patients who deferred initial treatment, survival at the end of 15 years was identical to that found in 77 men who did receive early treatment. If there was any question about the provocative implications of the observational study, the criticism of American activism in prostate cancer was made explicit by the Swedish trialist. He said, 'I think you overtreat many patients in the United States.'[2]

The only way to settle this important transnational controversy is to mount a concurrent comparison of the two policies—but this is easier said than done. A US controlled trial of treatment for prostate cancer was attempted in the 1970's. Although there was no difference in the 15-year survival in 61 men treated surgically, and in 50 who were not operated, the investigators admitted, 'there really weren't enough people [enrolled] to test the hypothesis that surgery can save lives.' A current trial has tried to enrol 1050 men; but after 3 years of effort, only 315 agreed to participate. Two urologists, who refused to participate in the study, were heard to say, '[We] can do without the trial . . . [we] can make inferences and study the case histories of our own patients to conclude that we are doing the right thing.' One practitioner declared, 'Everybody who's out there on the front line really knows [prostatectomy] works.'

The reluctance to admit the lack of hard evidence about the role of prostatectomy ensures that the controversy will not be settled easily. However, widespread screening of older men has revealed a surprisingly high prevalence of prostate cancer in the US.[2] The costs of aggressive surgical treatment to combat the newly recognised 'epidemic' are now enormous, and these economic pressures may force a showdown. 'True believers' may be forced by Mammon to put their faith to the test.

5

Humane limits
(1988)

If it's working, keep doing it.
If it's not working, stop doing it.
If you don't know what to do, don't do anything.
Advice to medical students[1]

Tyros quickly learn that the idealist's admonition, 'Don't just do something, stand there!' is easier said than done in the present era of action-oriented high-tech medicine. And, it becomes clear when they read a bit of history, current attitudes about interventions are not entirely unique. 'Doctors dressed up in one professional costume or another,' Lewis Thomas pointed out,[2] 'have been in busy practise since the earliest records of every culture on earth.' *Do* something! is a universal request at the onset of pain and suffering of illness—'healers' have responded with imagination and boundless enthusiasm (p. 1).

There was one relatively brief period of exception that began in the mid-19th century when some doctors questioned the wisdom of medicine's long tradition of undisciplined activism. Josef Skoda of Vienna spoke for many of these 'therapeutic nihilists' when he said,[3] 'While we can diagnose and describe disease, we dare not expect by any manner of means to cure it' (only God performs miracles, was the implication). Fildes' famous painting, 'The Doctor', depicting a physician sitting at the bedside of a dying child, provided a widely admired image of that period.[4] The doctor is shown leaning forward, chin cupped in hand, with a kindly, puzzled expression on his face—but doing nothing!

The therapeutic explosion following the Second World War did away with any notion that doctors would remain observers sitting passively at the bedside of the sick and dying. Miracles wrought by penicillin, streptomycin, polio vaccine and steroids provided convincing evidence that things would never be the same again: God-like therapeutic powers were now in the all-too-fallible hands of mortals. The newly-found capability to change the 'natural' course of events was evident, and strikingly so, in the new and rapidly expanding field of neonatal medicine. (One perceptive journalist described the remarkable new activities in a book entitled *Playing God in the Nursery.*)[5] Nonetheless, there is a strong undercurrent of unease about the achievements in neonatology.

Success, as measured by increased survival of neonates once considered pre-viable or hopelessly deformed, has come so quickly it is easy to forget that there is no clear consensus—even in the most affluent societies—about the allocation of available resources to modify pregnancy outcome. How much should be invested in the halfway technologies of medical rescue? How much in social intervention to reduce unfavourable outcome? (The dilemma is not unlike the one faced by a mountain town with a dangerous curve on its main road—the parable was quoted often by Sir Truby King, the founder of New Zealand's Plunket Society. Should the town post a fully-manned ambulance at the foot of the mountain, ready to rush crash victims to the hospital? Or should they build a guard rail on the outer rim of the curve to reduce the risk that autos will careen off the road?)

There is growing concern about the rapidly diminishing returns from the steady increase in manpower and material resources allocated for the acute care of the smallest and most seriously damaged infants.[6] In Australia, an often framed, but rarely expressed, question is now openly confronted:[7] Are some babies simply too small to be worth trying to save? At one institution in Melbourne the answer was 'Yes,' in 1987—infants weighing less than 800 gm were frequently not provided with full intensive care because to do so would constitute 'ineffective use of the institution's limited medical resources.'[8]

Parents also have doubts. Many are horrified to see their helpless, often curarised, fetus-like child rigged with tubes and wires connected to an array of flashing and beeping machines. The innumerable painful procedures carried out day after day to keep the fragile baby alive seem inhumane (and would be so labelled by the Royal Society for the Prevention of Cruelty to Animals if inflicted on a pet animal). 'Is it all worth it?' parents ask themselves. The question often refers to costs that extend well beyond those of medical concern. Many families have in mind the ephemeral price defined by Henry David Thoreau:[9] 'The cost of a thing is the amount of what I will call life which is required to be exchanged for it immediately or in the long run.'

(1997)

The progressive increase in survival of infants born very early in gestation has continued apace. Obstetricians now look to the most recent estimates of survival for guidance about termination of pregnancy when they are faced with the threatened birth of a fetal-infant at the threshold of viability.

A recent report of a 12-year, prospective, population-based survey of outcomes in the north of England has indicated a fairly sharp boundary at 24 weeks' gestation.[1] Survival to at least 1 year, of babies of 24–27 weeks' gestation in this cohort, increased steadily in the years 1983–1994. However, the viability of fetal-infants born before 24 weeks' gestation did not change; and most of the relatively few survivors in this category were found to be severely disabled. The British observers point out similar findings reported in Europe: 'no evidence of long term survival in babies born before 24 weeks' gestational age'. Yet, obstetricians in North America are aware that 'neonatal survival rates increase rapidly [between 23 and 24 weeks' gestation—ca 600–700 grams], varying from 10% to 50%;' and that disabilities among these survivors range from 20% to 35%.[2,3]

The British reviewers suspect that the apparent discrepancy in thresholds of viability on opposite sides of the Atlantic will be explained by differences in the demographic compositions of the at-risk populations. But the finding also fuels a suspicion that an explanation will be found in different attitudes and actions to prolong the lives of these borderline fetal-infants.

A comprehensive multinational study is now underway to develop an evidence-based framework for 'the development of ethical, clinical and public-policy guidelines for the care of very low birthweight infants.'[4] The comparison of the current range of deployment of resources for neonatal-rescue and the range of outcomes in different countries should provide a societal perspective of the choices now being made in efforts to breach the biological limits of human viability. In this age of pervasive technology, the broad examination of the state of the art may also provide an urgently needed reminder for the restraint advised by Jacques Ellul,[5] the famous French philosopher who was particularly interested in how technical means shape action. He concluded that: 'Human beings must agree not to do everything they are able to do.'

6

Intruding in private tragedies (1988)

The American system of bioethical committees...must be the
ultimate cop-out: An exercise in buck-passing...The most
important people in the negotiations, namely the baby and its
parents seem to have the least influence on the decisions.

J.E.S. Scott[1]

In the recent past, a treat-or-let-be decision after the birth of a very small
or seriously malformed baby was made quietly by the parents guided by
information provided by their doctor. Somewhere along the way from
then to now, and with increasing frequency, these private agonies have
been transformed into public spectacles. The sensational trial of Leonard
Arthur,[2] several years ago, on a charge of attempted murder was a revealing example of the noisy entry of new players on the neonatal scene.
Self-appointed moralists demonstrated that they were now prepared to
play a highly visible and pre-emptive role in treat-or-let-be deliberations.

Public opinion at the time of the trial at Leicester agreed with the
jury in rejecting the uninvited intrusion. A MORI poll[3] indicated that
86% (of 1 953 respondents) agreed that if a doctor, with parents' consent,
allowed a malformed newborn baby to die, he should not be found guilty
of murder. There was little support for doctors alone (4%) or law courts
(2%) to have a say whether a markedly handicapped baby lives or dies.
Notwithstanding public support for parents' primary role in these difficult decisions, the pleas of those directly involved seemed to be drowned
out in the cacophony of voices claiming to speak for the extremely small
or malformed neonate. Loud arguments about intervention are now made
frequently in court rooms, on printed pages, and in television broadcasts.
Melodramatic aspects of family tragedies are exploited shamelessly—
especially in the United States.

A warning about the oppressive influence of meddlers was issued
several years ago by the New York Court of Appeals.[4,5] In a case involving
parents who elected conservative rather than surgical treatment for their
infant born with major neural tube defects (spina bifida, hydrocephalus

and microcephaly), the court affirmed that 'a most private and most precious responsibility is vested in parents for the care of their child'. The ruling accepted the premise that the choice to forego surgery (after consultation with neurosurgeons, social worker and clergy) was made with love and thoughtfulness. A lawsuit to displace the primary responsibility of these parents was dismissed as an 'offensive action'.

The hospital-based 'infant bioethics committee'[6] is charged with the task of resolving inevitable disagreements that arise when trying to decide whether or not to forego life-sustaining treatment for a severely compromised neonate. On the surface, the democratic process does seem a reasonable way out of the ethical difficulties: After a full review of the facts, committee members from several disciplines vote by secret ballot. But this facile solution is an example of bioethical reductionism: It reduces complex ethical dimensions to simple processes and procedures. Churchill reminds us[7] that any decision, no matter how clearly justified in terms of ethical theory, must be persuasive to the person who is the moral agent. 'The assumption that ethical decision-making can be approached as a standard exercise,' he notes, 'ignores the vast range of human beliefs, sentiments and traditions which make the moral problem what it is, especially when these beliefs, sentiments and traditions resist precise articulation or formulation as problems to be solved.'

The shift of decision-making power from parents and personal doctors to infant bioethics committees results in a dilution of responsibility for decisions (pp. 53–57). The 'move is disturbingly close to the approach used by modern multinational corporations ('all but the most elementary decisions require information, specialised knowledge or experience of several or many people').[8] Malign consequences that have occurred as the result of decision-by-committee in the business world are well documented. Where is the evidence that would make us believe the fate of families with a malformed newly-born infant should be left to the 'vicissitudes of group dynamics among doctors, lawyers, ministers, ethicists and representatives of handicapped groups who bear no consequences' of the treatment decision?[9]

Who speaks up for the right to a humane and dignified death? A mother of a malformed infant who died at three months of age argued[10] that it is inappropriate for strangers to be part of the agonising treat-or-let-be decisions. Some events in life are simply so personal, so private that compassion and good sense demand they be left within the circle of family and family doctor. Parents, she advised, should be left to work out their enormous difficulties as best they can. Alone.

(1997)

Fourteen years after the agonising affair in Leicester (noted above), an equally wrenching life-and-death drama was enacted in the US. The

American incident took place in 1994 at East Lansing, Michigan, after a doctor's wife went into preterm labour at an estimated 25–26 weeks of gestation.[1] The staff neonatologist conferred with the parents before delivery, and explained that intensive measures would, very likely, be necessary to rescue the expected fetal-infant. Both parents feared that heroic intervention would subject their extremely premature baby to prolonged and unacceptable pain and suffering. They requested that resuscitation not be attempted at the time of birth.

A male infant was delivered several hours later by Caesarean section; gestational age was estimated at 25 weeks, birthweight was 780 grams, and the newborn was described as 'lifeless and dark.' A physician's assistant intubated the baby, began mechanical ventilation, and brought him to the neonatal intensive care unit where he was placed on a ventilator. When the parents came to the unit and saw that intensive intervention was underway, they asked to be left alone with their son. The professional staff left the room. A short time later a nurse reported that the father had disconnected the ventilator and the mother was holding her moribund baby. The staff elected 'not to intervene at this time;' and the infant died a short time later, while in his mother's arms.

The father was arrested and charged with manslaughter. In January 1995, he was tried and quickly acquitted on the first ballot taken by the jurors.[2] A law student, who served as the jury foreman, later said that the disenfranchisement of the parents, disclosed in the trial, left her frightened at the thought of ever having children.

Modern medicine's fearsome power, recognised by the Michigan jury, is not confined to the field of neonatology. For example, one survey of the hospital experiences of seriously-ill patients revealed that doctors frequently failed to comply with their patients' express wishes not to be resuscitated.[3] A programme was devised to improve communication about the preference to forego cardiopulmonary resuscitation. The experimental plan was tested in a randomised trial (p. 182). The hopes for improvement were not realised: there was no important increase in physician–patient agreement about 'do not resuscitate' orders. The disappointed researchers were left to wonder 'what elements of context and culture of health care might have to be altered, to ease suffering...and avoid inappropriate treatment?' This anxiety about present-day medicine's never-say-die zeal is completely justified. Note, for instance, that the policy for mandatory resuscitation of cardiac arrest by the emergency medical service in one American city,[4] excludes only persons who have been decapitated, those who exhibit rigor mortis, or have signs of physical decomposition!

7

The glut of information (1989)

It seems to me that we should, for an experimental period of
a year, declare a moratorium on the appending of authors'
names and the names of hospitals to articles in medical journals. . . . If dissemination of information is the reason why
papers are submitted for publication, there will be no falling
off in the numbers offered.

J.B. Healy[1]

Any suspicion that there has been a dramatic increase in the number of
medical articles published each year is easily confirmed—simply weigh
the annual volumes of *Index Medicus*.[2] (It has been estimated that the
biomedical literature is expanding at a compound rate of 6–7 per cent
each year.)[3] Moreover, the overwhelming increase has been accompanied
by growth in the numbers of authors listed at the head of each paper.[4,5]
How can readers cope with this unprecedented glut of data—the flood
of text, numbers, tables and graphs that gushes forth from the word
processors of a growing army of busy medical writers?

'As writers become more numerous,' Oliver Goldsmith once observed,[6]
'it is natural for readers to become more indolent.' However, present-day
consumers of medical information must become more, rather than less
attentive in the face of the communication overload. It is clear that all
published articles must be approached with practised caution, for,
it turns out, a surprisingly high proportion of reported studies are
methodologically flawed. In one review of 4500 biomedical papers
published between 1950 and 1978, 80 per cent were found to be methodologically deficient.[7] There is little evidence that the situation has
improved in the years since that survey.[8] Editors of medical journals on
both sides of the Atlantic[8,10] are now quite disturbed about a patent
failure of the time-honoured peer review process to control the quality
of published information. 'There seems to be,' Drummond Rennie, editor
of the *Journal of the American Medical Association*, opined,[9] 'no study too
fragmented, no hypothesis too trivial, no literature citation too biased or

too egotistical, no design too warped, no methodology too bungled, no presentation of results too inaccurate and too contradictory, no analysis too self-serving, no argument too circular, no conclusion too trifling or too unjustified, and no grammar and syntax too offensive for a paper to end up in print.' It seems, to put it mildly, the crisis in confidence concerning quality control is very serious.

Four differing perceptions of the current refereeing process have been identified:[11] 'the sieve (peer review screens worthy from unworthy submissions), the switch (a persistent author can eventually get anything published, but peer review determines where), the smithy (papers are pounded into new and better shapes between the hammer of peer review and the anvil of editorial standards), and the shot in the dark (peer review is essentially unpredictable and unreproducible and hence, in effect, random).' It is remarkable that there is little more than opinion to support these characterisations of the gate-keeping process which plays such a critical role in the operation of today's huge medical research enterprise ('peer review is the linch pin of science').[9] There have been very few carefully crafted studies of the process. Bailar and Paterson are quite right to point out a paradox here: the judges of rigour, quality, and innovation in manuscripts submitted for publication do not, it seems, apply to their own work the standards they use in evaluating the work of others.

The implied warranty of methodological rigour in articles that appear in highly regarded journals is disturbingly weak. Readers have no choice; they must develop their own coping strategies if they are to make sense out of even the most highly touted printed information that passes before their eyes day after day. Fortunately, help has been made available. David Sackett and his fellow clinical epidemiologists have provided flow charts of guides to assist in a critical read of the medical literature.[12] They have given doctors an efficient plan: It separates the 'wheat from the chaff' quickly and reduces the chance of engulfment by endless reports of innovations in diagnosis, prognosis, and therapy.

After publication, most articles sink without a trace (or they turn up later, only as self-citations). It has been suggested[13] that citation analysis (the number of times a published paper is cited, subsequently, by co-workers) might provide readers with an objective measure of lasting impact and, one would hope, the quality of individual publications. For example, we might expect that well designed and properly executed studies are cited more often than flawed exercises. Although a trend associating rigour with citation has been found in one study,[14] the correlation was weak. Citation count was not, it seemed, a reliable indicator of the quality of an individual paper's study design. Although the results of the study were somewhat disappointing, the experience did call attention to three issues which cry out for further exploration:[15] what characteristics should be taken into account in judging the quality of a research report, how shall this quality be measured, and what use shall be made of the defined and measured quality?

An international conference was convened in 1989,[16] to examine the problem of peer review in biomedical publication. The organisers stressed responsibility, as it applies to authors and editors, and the improvement of quality control over the entire review procedure (e.g. Should the names of authors and institutions be withheld from referees?[17,18] Should data and conclusions be withheld to shift judgmental emphasis from examination of results to increased probing of investigative methods?).[19] The conferees were prepared to advise scrapping the peer review process entirely, if research should confirm current fears about inadequacy of the traditional format.

Rennie quotes the view of the illustrious pathologist, Rudolph Virchow, voiced in a simpler age. In his *Archiv für pathologische Anatomie and Physiologie* the great man said: 'In my journal, anyone can make a fool of himself.'

(1997)

The Second International Congress on Peer Review was convened in 1993.[1] When the attendees were queried about a number of topics, the majority of respondents agreed there was a need to investigate the prevalence of scientific fraud. The topic of misconduct also surfaced in an invited address to the Congress by Judson;[2] he recognised that the review process was 'inherently threatened by corruption.' The basic contradiction in a review by peers, he noted, arises from the fact that persons most qualified to judge the worth of a paper submitted by an investigator, are 'precisely those who are that scientist's closest competitors.'

The most encouraging development growing out of the increased interest in the review process is the founding of Locknet[3]—a network of groups examining all facets of the topic (including that of scientific integrity). However, current dilemmas may be rendered moot by the explosive development of electronic publishing. This revolution may transform scientific publication so completely, that it may become unrecognisable in the very near future. The dramatic change may turn out to be a welcome advance, Judson opined, if it 'will open up the processes by which scientists judge each others work, making them less anonymous, capricious, rigid, subject to abuse, and more thorough, responsible, and accountable.'

However, we should not minimise the daunting problem of evaluating the validity of evidence set out in the electronically-available glut of raw data, and in assertions, rebuttals, suggestions, criticisms, revisions, and so on. There is a danger that lurks in this new Age of Information,

Roszack warns,[4] '[It] makes every computer around us what the religious relics were in the Age of Faith—emblems of salvation.' Shenk has also warned[5] about dire consequences of what he terms 'information obesity.' 'Just as fat has replaced starvation as [the] number one dietary concern,' he opines, 'information overload has replaced information scarcity as an important new emotional, social, and political problem.'

8

Betting on specified horses
(1989)

A science does not truly become mature until it develops a predictive capability.

Peter Medawar[1]

The recent death of Sir Peter Medawar reminds us of how much we owe him for many enduring contributions to biology, and, in particular, for his philosophic arguments about the nature of scientific thought. A series of lectures about the epistemology of science, delivered by him almost 30 years ago, is specially memorable.[2] In those talks, he characterised a scientist as, first and foremost, a questioner of received beliefs. He pointed to Francis Galton's *Statistical Inquiries Into the Efficacy of Prayer*[3] as one of the clearest displays of the critical temper of science. (Galton examined the longevity of royal families—something prayed for on a national scale. He found that, if anything, royalty fared worse than did people of humbler birth. The mean age at death of 97 male members of royal houses was 64 years—a shorter life span, on average, than that attained by the clergy, lawyers, the medical profession, and seven other classes of British men.)

Medawar then argued that the popular conception of the scientist (as a critic, a sceptic, one who is intolerant or contemptuous of conventional beliefs) is not far off the mark; but the image is not complete. The exposure of error, he noted, merely clears obstacles from the path of progress—it does not propel science forward. To prove that pigs cannot fly is not to devise a machine that does so.

Clearly, there is another side to the scientific enterprise. In medicine, most particularly, we are aware of the need to maintain a delicate balance between demolition and construction. The operation has been likened to that of continually rebuilding a huge ship in the middle of the ocean—dismantlers of the superannuated bits must be careful not to get too far ahead of the builders. Moreover, the 'shipwrights' must have a vision of the future. Indeed, when a claim is made that completed projects are 'seaworthy,' medical scientists are required to make very specific predictions about natural events that have not yet occurred.

The hypothetico-deductive scheme of thought, Medawar noted, places a premium on the element of prior expectation when examining new events. The scheme allows for a running adjustment of a predictive model by the process of negative feedback: If events take place as forecast, the model need not be altered, but modification is mandatory when the prediction is clearly wrong.

Tukey discussed the prediction issue[4] from the point of view of statisticians who are asked, for the sake of future patients, to help wring as much as possible, say, out of a set of data obtained in a therapeutic trial. He warned about the interpretive problems that arise under these circumstances. For example, in a *clinical inquiry* an intervention is used in the hope that it will help some class of patients, not specified in advance. Massive amounts of data are collected and the results are analysed for each of many subclasses of patients (by age, sex, previous medical history, prognosis, symptoms. . .). Separate analyses for different outcomes may also be requested. The large body of information is obtained with few, if any, specific a priori questions in mind. But when we ask many questions and concentrate on the most favourable answers this leads inexorably to an increased likelihood of stumbling on misleading coincidences. (Keep in mind the Alice-in-Wonderland principle: If you don't know where you are going, almost any road will take you there!) Moreover, we can expect no help from statistical arithmetic. None of the formulations take into account the history of the investigator's mind-set. For example, significance tests make no distinction between the credibility of prior hypotheses and that of data-suggested associations.[5]

The strength of evidence obtained in blurred exercises should be distinguished from a *focused* clinical trial. In the latter study both the class of patients and the expected outcome are clearly specified in the study protocol. Louis and co-workers use the phrase 'investigative intent' to describe the few questions of primary interest set out in specific detail before study data are collected.[6] 'The results of broad data dredging should be given less scientific weight,' is their wise advice. 'Fishing expeditions' in the pool of information collected in clinical inquiries are helpful in exploring the dimensions of interesting questions, but we would do well to insist on focused trials for reasonably trustworthy conclusions.

It should not be surprising that we need to make specific predictions if we are to make sense about cause-and-effect in the outcome of variable events. The requirement is demanded regularly in everyday life to help distinguish between chance and meaningful relationships. For instance, the story is told of a visiting Indian Rajah who was invited to Ascot Down for the horse races. He declined, saying, 'It is already known to me that one horse can run faster than another.' When it was explained that before the race begins gamblers bet that one specific horse will win, the Prince went to the racetrack—eagerly.

(1997)

Tukey's warning to researchers, 20 years ago, is still relevant: Resist the temptation to collect endless numbers of observations and measurements when precise forecasts have not been set out before the data are collected. The compulsion to record everything should be called the 'last-bus-out-of-town syndrome,' because it is so like the approach to data collection in the early space projects. The scientists and engineers 'planned each mission with the fear that it's the last bus out of town and everybody's got to get aboard with every conceivable instrument.'[1]

On the other hand (as noted above), opportunities for a reasonable number of 'fishing expeditions' seeking unpredicted associations should not be overlooked, so long as these are clearly labelled as hypothesis-generating operations. And a 'double-pond' approach (to separate data used for 'prediction' from another set used as a 'test') is a useful way to structure these *post hoc* analyses. For example, Zupancic and co-workers recently conducted a survey of a number of determinants that might influence parents' decisions to enrol their children in controlled trials.[2] The sample responses were randomised into two equal parts: one half was used to generate a multiple regression model, and the validity of the model was tested in the second half of the dataset.

The principle, again, is straightforward: 'The ultimate standard for the success of an idea in science is the sustained agreement between prediction and result.[3] The important word here is 'sustained,' because in clinical research, this is often the weakest link in the chain of proof. There is very little enthusiasm for carrying out much-needed replications, because they are dismissed, too often, as 'unoriginal' work. But seasoned reporters who comment on the medical scene have come to understand the situation. 'The first paper was intriguing,' Kolata has written.[4] 'With the next three you begin to become more concerned. Now you would like the real answer.'

9

Begin with 'If . . .'
(1989)

Clocks will go as they are set, but man, irregular man, is never constant, never certain.

Thomas Otway (1652–1685)

Some critics of randomised clinical trial (RCT) methodology charge that the approach is of 'limited value in the resolution of strongly-held conflicting views about new therapies.'[1] Among other perceived shortcomings, the complainers direct attention to inconsistency of results—the wide variation in outcomes when the trials are replicated. An example of the contrariety surfaced in 1986 when a large-scale RCT reported that, unlike favourable results in previous small trials, phenobarbitone prophylaxis in neonates was associated with an unexpected increase in the risk of intracranial haemorrhage.[2]

Why, one wonders, has the RCT been singled out for this vote of no confidence concerning external validity (generalisability of results)? Random order of assignments in a treatment comparison trial is intended to improve the chances for internal consistency: prognostic characteristics of enrolled patients are represented equally in each of the treatment groups. There is, it must be recognised, an important distinction between 'patients enrolled,' 'patients eligible,' and 'patients available;' they are subsets of the 'parent population'—the total number of patients in a defined class. The allotment precaution has no influence on the likelihood of drawing a representative sample of participants from that parent population—the intended beneficiaries of information acquired in the trial.

The 'generality of the answer' (Sir Austin Bradford Hill's felicitous phrase[3]) in all formats of clinical investigation is hemmed in by questions about the representativeness of patients enrolled in a given study. Participants are not, by any stretch of the imagination, probability samples picked out from the parent population under strict rules of random sampling. Selection bias of one kind or another is clearly unavoidable. The inherent characteristics of patients that influence their systematic choices of doctors and hospitals, patterns of referral by physicians, special interests in 'centres of excellence,' admitting practices (when hospitals are crowded, only the most severely affected patients with a disease of interest are admitted; in slack periods, patients with relatively mild forms of the same disorder are hospitalised), differing financial and geographic access to diagnostic tests that identifies patients as eligible for clinical study, etc., are but a few in a long list of biasing influences that bring about an irreproducible sorting of patients.[4] As a result, the characteristics of patients available for study may vary widely between (and within) institutions from one period of time to another.

An additional opportunity for selection bias opens wide at the time of the consent-to-enrol step in clinical studies. Since we depend on patients who give their consent freely, enrolees are, by definition, a self-selected sample of those eligible to participate. It is hazardous to assume that the volunteer/participants are typical representatives of the available population (much less the parent population) which includes eligible patients who refuse to be enrolled in the study.[5]

Sackett and his co-workers have cited[6] a revealing example of the 'volunteer/participant problem' that was identified in a large-scale randomised trial of screening for breast cancer. As compared with controls enrolled in the trial, there was a striking reduction in breast cancer mortality among women (over age 50) who had routine mammography and breast examination. The mortality from other causes of death was identical in the two arms of the screening trial, confirming internal consistency (random allotment was successful in setting up comparable groups of women in the experimental and control groups). At the recruiting stage of the trial two-thirds of the eligible women were willing to participate, one-third refused. This experience provided an opportunity to compare volunteer/participants with refusers in regard to causes of death for which they were not screened. The subset of women who volunteered for breast cancer screening died from other (non-breast-cancer) causes at a rate about one-half that experienced by the refusers; volunteer/participants did very well, it seemed, with diseases for which they were never screened and were never (on this account) treated! 'Volunteers for screening,' Sackett's group warns, 'are generally a strange and healthy lot, and we cannot generalise from them to other patients.'

Similar questions about external validity arise when doctors manipulate the recruitment of patients in formal trials. The disturbance concerning enrolment in the international extracranial-to-intracranial bypass randomised trial to prevent ischaemic stroke is another example of the kinds of difficulties that turn up.[7] It has been estimated that 50–70% of eligible patients, in 71 centres throughout the world, were not included in the trial because consent for randomisation was not granted by referring doctors or their patients (many of the refusers were treated surgically outside of the formal trial by the trial surgeons). At the end of the trial it was found that surgical intervention in enrolled patients was ineffective; but there is simply no way to know (and statistical arithmetic is not helpful in deciding) what the results would have been if all the eligible patients had been enrolled.

Donald Mainland has warned[8] that concluding statements in all clinical studies ought to begin with *'If'* and their verbs should be in the subjunctive mood: *'If* this were a strictly random sample from a population completely defined in all relevant respects, the inferences would be. . . .' Clinical studies, it needs to be understood, are subject to substantially more variability than is indicated by standard statistical tests and confidence intervals.[9] 'The only way to learn something about the safety of our numerical findings,' Mainland once warned (p. 166),[10] 'is by more extensive exploration under other conditions, and at other times.'

When is it safe to move from 'comparative trials' to 'acceptance for everyday use' of a new treatment? There comes a time when we must take courage in hand even though all suspicions about the generality of the answer have not been put to rest. The US Food and Drug Administration requires[11] 'Phase IV Postmarketing studies' to determine the incidence of adverse reactions of a new drug and its impact on morbidity and mortality when the new agent is first deployed in the field. But 'postmarketing' monitoring of innovations is often honoured in the breach. Reports of untoward effects are largely anecdotal—lonely numerators looking for faintly visible denominators.

Given the uncertainties about wide extrapolation of results after any and all formal clinical studies, it makes sense to consider a graded approach to the release of a promising innovation for everyday use. Instead of country-wide release, as at present, in a step-wise plan new treatment would be made available in only one city or other circumscribed region in order to monitor closely the initial field experience with, now, unselected patients. (In commerce, this kind of 'test marketing' within a manageable geographical unit is considered a prudent way to disclose unexpected complications when a new product is first put up for public sale.) Jennett's proposal[12] for developing predictive models to assess the limits of utility of technological packages used in the clinical management of specific disorders in different geographic sites might be adapted for use in a plan of stepwise release of innovations.

(1997)

David Moore, an American statistician, quotes[1] Samuel Johnson ('You don't have to eat the whole ox to know the meat is tough') to introduce the essential idea behind sampling. But in examining the part to obtain information about the whole, he emphasises, the method used to obtain representative 'bites' is crucial.

Unfortunately, statisticians have had remarkably little success in convincing researchers that Mainland's caveat about this issue (*'If* this were a strictly random sample. . . .') describes a serious limit to the extrapolation of results obtained in virtually every clinical study. Ellenberg recently charged[2] that '[T]he scientific community has not . . . accepted the necessity for critical assessment of the method of sample selection in the planning and execution of studies, as a fundamental underpinning of observational and experimental studies.' The failing is obvious, he adds 'in the plethora of research studies receiving funding, being published in peer-reviewed journals, and influencing future studies that may be reporting entirely spurious associations.'

Ellenberg makes a strong plea for increased attention to the potential damage caused by selection bias in many study designs. (As already noted, selective enrolment in the international by-pass trial to prevent ischaemic stroke[3] created questions about the generalisation of results that simply cannot be answered). 'The notion that "this is the best we can do,"' he argues, 'does not appear to me to be the appropriate marching orders, if the best we can do is mediocre.'

10

Archie's scepticism (1989)

My colleagues, in their devotion to their patients, evoke my admiration, but also remind me of [the demands of families that "nothing be left undone"]. I hope clinicians in the future will abandon the 'margin of the impossible' and settle for "reasonable probability."

Archie Cochrane[1]

No one had better insight concerning doctors' phobic fears of concurrent controls in clinical studies than Archie Cochrane. The news of his recent death triggered another read of a well-thumbed copy of Cochrane's famous monograph, *Effectiveness and Efficiency*.[1] In it he tells a revealing and wonderfully human story about the hang-up that plays such an obstructive role in the design and in the conduct of formal clinical investigation.

When debate about number-of-coronary-care-units-needed was heating up, Mather and co-workers mounted the now well-known controlled clinical trial to compare treatment of ischaemic heart disease at-home vs in-hospital.[2] Prejudgment-bias was illustrated beautifully, Cochrane wrote, in an incident that occurred a few months after the trial began. Interim results showed a slightly higher death rate for hospital-treated than for home-treated patients. Someone reversed the figures and showed them to a CCU-enthusiast who immediately called for an end to the trial: 'It is unethical,' the advocate said, 'and must be stopped at once.' When, however, the pro-CCU doctor was shown the numbers correctly put, he could not be persuaded to condemn care in CCUs as unethical!

In the years after publication of the story in *Effectiveness and Efficiency*, Cochrane frequently used the example in his lectures. At the end of the talks, he was almost invariably approached by a doctor in the audience who would say, in effect, 'But surely, Professor Cochrane, if you yourself had acute myocardial ischaemia you would want to be treated in hospital.' After years of enduring this sort of disparaging commentary, Cochrane did, at one time, suffer a myocardial incident. He could hardly

wait to inform all callers, 'Be sure to tell everyone you know that I was
treated at home.'

It is interesting to see how prescient Cochrane was in pointing to the
exact area of misunderstanding that would continue to plague efforts to
find out which treatments are effective and how efficiently they are
applied. In the experience with the mixed reaction to interim results, he
saw, correctly, the seeds of a growing controversy. For example, one moral
philosopher now declares that 'randomised clinical trials as presently
conducted are unethical.'[3] There is an irresolvable conflict, the philosopher contends, between a doctor's 'therapeutic obligation' (always to
prescribe the best treatment known) and continued participation in a
trial as soon as interim results show that a trend has developed in favour
of one of the compared treatments. And this misunderstanding among
ethicists about the problem of making sure predictions of the outcomes
of interventions in individual patients seems difficult to dispel.[4]

The overinterpretation of early trends in clinical trials reveals a
curious lack of understanding about biological variation. The naive view
is as unreal as an expectation that perfectly matched horses must run
exactly even for an entire race. Surely no bettor could convince officials
to stop the race as soon as his/her horse took the lead. Nonetheless,
the debates between moralists and trialists seems to be increasing in
intensity. Archie Cochrane's sane voice (and humour!) will be missed in
the uphill struggle to explain the ethical propriety of a planned approach
to the problem of medical uncertainty.[5]

Another theme came through loud and clear in the 1971 monograph
and it resounds to the present day. 'I believe,' Cochrane wrote, 'that cure
is rare while the need for care is widespread, and that the pursuit of cure
at all costs may restrict the supply of care.' He came to this view the
hard way: in experiences as a prisoner of war in German hands for four
years. While in a *Dulag* in Salonika and later in Elsterholst, Cochrane was
often the only senior medical officer trying to render care to thousands of
his fellow prisoners with little or no drugs and medical equipment.

One incident at Elsterholst (not noted in the monograph) made a
searing impression. All the POWs with tuberculosis (most with advanced disease) of all nationalities were herded together in one site at
this camp. Although there were facilities that made it possible to treat
patients with bed-rest, pneumothorax and pneumo-peritoneum, no pain
relieving drugs were provided by the Germans. Cochrane remembered
one night when a dying patient in excruciating pain screamed without
let up for hours. Unable to provide any relief, Cochrane put his arms
around the man and hugged him tightly—the screaming stopped almost
immediately and the man died peacefully several hours later in
Cochrane's arms.

In the Salonika *Dulag* there were 20 000 prisoners whose medical
needs were served in a ramshackle hospital with some aspirin, antacid,

and skin antiseptic. For a considerable time, Cochrane was the only doctor. The prisoners were fed 600 calories a day, all had diarrhoea, and there were severe epidemics of typhoid, diphtheria, other infections, jaundice and sand-fly fever. More than 300 of the POWs developed pitting oedema above the knee. Under the best of conditions, Cochrane noted, one would have expected hundreds to die of diphtheria alone in the absence of specific therapy. As it happened, there were only four deaths, of which three were due to gunshot wounds inflicted by the Germans.

The amazing result convinced Cochrane of the relative unimportance of therapy in comparison with the recuperative powers of the human body. In the midst of the experience in the *Dulag*, he asked the Germans for more doctors to help him cope with the fantastic problems. 'No!,' he was told, 'Doctors are superfluous.' The young Cochrane was furious and wrote a poem about his frustration,

> Superfluous Doctors—what a phrase to rouse
> Dulled prison fires to flicker the muse
> And build a brave new world. There would be
> No famines, wars, or other acts of God
> To break the Peace on Earth. No! Man would turn
> From wanton killing of his cousin's kin
> To face his very foes, and Science, Art
> With Labour in ally, would fight and kill
> Want and its fears, disease, its very roots,
> Squalor and filth and loneliness and pain;
> And then let doctors quit the centre stage
> To usher in the prophylactic age.

> But death was near and hunger, and prisoners' dreams were rare
> The doctor in Salonika sat down and tore his hair.

Later, Archie Cochrane wondered if his captors were wise or cruel; they were, he concluded, certainly right.

(1997)

A retrospective examination[1] of a debate in the 1970s about medicine's shortcomings, has documented the fact that Archie Cochrane's arguments were among the most widely heard and the most influential. '*Effectiveness and Efficiency*' was cited in 430 papers in the first 18 years after publication in 1972,[2] and the monograph was translated into French, Spanish, Italian and Polish. In Cochrane's reformist view, evidence from randomised trials was essential to inform rational choices made by health policy experts, by practitioners, and by patients. In another influential paper published in 1979,[3] he criticised the profession for its repeated failures to conduct timely systematic reviews of accumulating clinical evidence. He wrote: 'It is surely a great criticism of our profession that we have not organised a critical summary, by speciality or subspeciality, updated periodically, of all relevant randomised controlled trials.'

This second jeremiad also had an important impact on medical thought and action. And Archie lived to see the first response to his prodding: In 1987, the year before he died, he referred to the first systematic reviews of controlled trials in pregnancy and childbirth as 'a real milestone in the history of randomised trials and in the evaluation of care'.[4]

A group of collaborators around the world recognised the need for a practical mechanism to expand the scope of updated overviews to encompass all of health care.[5] It also became clear that the explosive electronic revolution could provide the practical means to disseminate these reviews world-wide. When the Research and Development programme of the National Health Service (NHS) was created in 1991 to develop an evaluative culture across the NHS, an opportunity arose to 'get to grips with Archie Cochrane's agenda.'[6] Accordingly, a centre named in his honour was established in Oxford in October 1992. The goal of this UK Cochrane Centre was 'to collaborate with others in building and maintaining a core database of systematic up-to-date reviews of randomised controlled trials of health care, and to arrange for these reviews to be readily accessible through various electronic media.' The International Cochrane Collaboration, now consisting of centres throughout the world, is an eponymous and altogether fitting tribute to the man who did so much to convince clinical medicine to transform itself into an evidence-based discipline.[7] ◆

11

Arbitrary vs discretionary decisions
(1990)

> We must recognise that even when clinicians make decisions
> based on the best evidence available, their own ethical, moral
> and religious values influence their medical decision-making.[1]

The Nuer tribe of East Africa is said to be unable to cope with defective newborn infants.[2] They classify strange neonates as hippopotamuses, mistakenly born to human parents. The 'animals' are put gently into a river, their 'natural habitat.' Nuer infants are not killed; the tribe says, in effect, we merely do what is proper for young hippos. The moral code of the Nuer, which prohibits the taking of a tribe member's life, emerges unscathed in this solution to an ancient question about newly-born babies: What are the conditions for full membership in the family and community?

A Nuer-like end result was achieved in developed countries, when most babies were delivered at home. Midwives and doctors, when on the family's territory, were acutely aware of the immediate and long-term social consequences of their acts. They rarely made attempts to rescue a very small or a malformed infant. Within the privacy of the home, the early deaths of flawed babies were often reported as 'stillborn.'

Until fairly recently, neonatal deaths were seen as the 'expected' reproductive losses—similar in every way to the large initial mortality in all species. More specifically, it seemed inhumane to prolong the lives of seriously compromised babies. The metamorphosis of a newborn infant from biological creation to social being and family member took place only when nurturing care was provided by the family. Few parents, in the past were willing to place the interest of a newborn child with significant biological imperfections ahead of all others in the family.[3] There was a fairly general, but silent, understanding that the newborn infant had only a tentative claim to full rights of family membership.

It is a matter of some interest that a gradual shift in perspective and in action took place when decisions about the care of marginal infants were taken over by well-meaning doctors, and early nurturing care was provided in medical settings. For example, when the campaign to rescue prematurely-born infants was started by French obstetricians in the third quarter of the last century, the small 'weaklings' were transferred to special facilities for expert care.[4] Here skilled nurses provided warmth (in newly-designed incubators), cleanliness, careful feeding, and attentive care to minimise exertion of the weak babies. If favourable conditions for survival are provided, the caretakers reasoned, those infants 'meant' to survive would do so. This focus on *infant's* outcome, away from social impact on the family, was the beginning of a change in viewpoint that has persisted to the present day.

For many years there was resistance to the systematic approach for the care of 'weaklings.'[5] Many observers had serious doubts about the advisability of making extraordinary efforts to keep marginally-viable newborn infants alive. Although it might be praiseworthy to try to save these new lives, they argued, the efforts should be condemned as short-sighted. At the turn of the century, caretakers were urged to recognise that standing behind each of the feeble infants there was, very often, a family problem, ultimately a community problem, poverty, bad housing and associations, ignorance of the ways and means of making a clean and healthy life on scant means.

The explosive development of neonatal/perinatal medicine and escalation of intensive treatment of babies on the margins of intact viability, during the past few decades, have re-ignited earlier questions about child-centred measurements of outcome. There is renewed concern about the consequences of rescuing seriously compromised newborn infants without regard for the social circumstances of the family. The dilemma is now magnified several times over because the machinery of rescue has made it possible to keep ever more fragile infants alive who have an ever larger need for on-going medical and social support. For each increment of success in prolonging the lives of the smallest infants, the cost in resources has mounted dramatically.

How should decisions be made to initiate all-out modern treatment for the most costly infants (under 1 kg birthweight)?[6] We are largely ignorant of the relative impact of death (as compared with survival) of these smallest infants on families in poor circumstances, in single-parent families, after unwanted pregnancy, in families with drug-addicted parents, etc. The area of uncertainty might be narrowed if we could marshall the courage needed to submit some of the hard questions about decision-making to formal evaluation.[7] For a start, we might ask: Do arbitrary decisions at the time of impending birth of the smallest babies (presumption to initiate all-out treatment in most cases) result in improved long-term social outcomes in affected families, as compared with discretionary decisions (after discussion with parents, and based on their wishes, initiate either all-out treatment or non-invasive supportive care)? In order to explore a question with family status as the primary outcome of interest, it is not enough to examine the condition of families of infants who survive. Long-term social outcome in families in which the infant did *not* survive now becomes relevant.

Families and communities need to be thoroughly convinced of the social effectiveness of unbridled medical salvage. A direct comparison of the social consequences of carrying out either parents' wishes or doctors' orders is very threatening to conventional wisdom. It draws attention away from the professional question (How many neonatologists are needed?[8]) and focuses on the question of public interest (How many neonatologists are wanted?).

(1997)

Public concern about the level of investment of resources for neonatal rescue has increased as the costs of the activity have mounted. And loud questions are now asked about equality in the provision of overall medical care, taking into account the *competing* claims of individuals, families, and communities. Williams has made a timely plea[1] for the development of *evidence-based ethics* to guide judgements about care: factored decisions that are weighted to reflect the marginal social value of health gains to different people. The quantitative approach, he proposes, 'might help us develop a notion of "statistical compassion" (the ability to sympathise with the plight of the unfortunate but anonymous many) to help counteract the excesses of individual compassion (sympathy for the unfortunate but identifiable individual) which results in such severe inequity at present.'

The myopic never-say-die preoccupation of today's rescue industry brings to mind the apocryphal story about the man who went to a psychiatrist and complained, 'My brother is crazy; he thinks he's a chicken.' 'Why doesn't your family do something about it?' the doctor asked. 'We can't,' was the hapless reply, 'we need the eggs.'

12

Bioengineering
(1990)

Engineering is the art of directing the great sources of power
in nature for the use and convenience of man.

Thomas Tredgold[1]

In defence of unrestrained inquiry in the basic sciences, an atomic
physicist argued[2] that 'Science simply operates on the faith that knowledge is good and ignorance is something to overcome. You can't really
vindicate this faith empirically, it is a faith,' he said; then he hinted at
approval from a higher authority by citing the biblical injunction, 'Let
there be light.' The argument reflects a romantic view that sees a sharp
difference between the mission of scientists (they seek merely to understand the world) and the programme of actors in applied fields (the
engineers and physicians who labour to change it).

No such disengagement between inquiry and action was envisioned at
the very beginning of the scientific revolution in the seventeenth century.
Francis Bacon predicted[3] that organised scientific research would
increase human power to control the environment. In *Discourse on
Method*,[4] Descartes explained that use of his new principles when examining the natural world (resolution of complex problems into simpler
elements or component parts) would generate 'knowledge that will be
of much utility in this life.' The new mode of science, he said, will
'make ourselves masters and possessors ... of nature.' Descartes emphasised that his 'mechanical philosophy' (the analysis of all animal and
human functions by reducing them to machine-like actions) would have
many practical consequences for medicine.[5] He predicted the eventual
elimination of the 'illnesses of the body as well of the mind.'

The enormous success of more than 350 years of unrestrained scientific inquiry and engineering action, has been acclaimed by most, but not
all, social critics. For example, anxieties about the impacts of biotechnology are now much like the fears about the unrestricted applications in
atomic physics that have now made it possible not only to change the
world but to destroy it completely. A philosopher recently examined the

new interventions made possible by the remarkable progress in genetics and asked,[6] 'Are human beings obliged to keep their biological foundation intact, or must they manipulate the natural base?'

We are, in fact, busily engaged in manipulating our biological foundation. Nothing demonstrates the new power over basic biological processes so convincingly as the modern control of human reproduction.[7] We have to shake ourselves to realise that in an amazingly short time, the levers of power which control humankind's game of reproductive roulette have passed from the goddess of chance into the hands of the medical profession—antenatal and neonatal doctors are fast becoming an effective corps of biological and social engineers.

Pauly has traced[8] the modern revival of Descartes' interest in the control of life to developments in the late nineteenth century. The rekindling took place 100 years ago in the experimental laboratories of a number of biologists who adopted an expansive view of science and its power. They began to think of themselves and their work in the context of engineering. Jacques Loeb was the first to proclaim the ideal of biologist as engineer; he carried out his most important work in experimental biology within this conceptual framework. In 1890, Loeb told the physicist, Ernst Mach, 'the idea is now hovering before me that man himself can act as a creator, even in living Nature, forming it eventually to his will.'

Loeb had accepted Mach's faith in the ethical values inherent in research and he adopted the physicist's belief in the fundamental unity of science and technology. Science, Mach opined, is a human effort to cope with the environment. From 1890 to 1915, Loeb was the principal spokesman for what Pauly terms, the 'engineering point of view' in biology. The interest in controlling biological processes led Loeb in 1899 to his most notable achievement, the induction of artificial parthenogenesis in unfertilised eggs of the sea urchin. This startling modification of normal reproduction convinced him about the transformative potential of science. The technical success led him to argue confidently that biology in the twentieth century should be organised around engineering aims. Loeb began to make strong claims for the power to control life: His 'engineer in biology' was a man of action who weighed the importance of new concepts on the basis of their potential to rule over Nature.

Loeb's outlook slowly shifted in the years 1910 to 1918 from hopes for the power of biologists as agents of change, to a belief that scientists should observe biological phenomena passively and try to see the hidden mechanisms that underlie them. But the success of his earlier promotion of the engineering ideal is seen in the biotechnical innovations created by those who followed him. For example, Pauly reports that in 1930 Gregory Pincus decided that 'Loeb stopped too soon.' Pincus began to experiment with methods to control reproduction and, in 1956, perfected

the oral contraceptive. The far-reaching practical consequences of Pincus'
accomplishment fulfilled Loeb's earlier vision of an activist biology that
would achieve mastery over Nature.

In recent years, the need has become more pressing to make a clear
distinction between scientific activity (the search for understanding in
matters concerning human procreation), and medical engineering (the
application of that new knowledge in the form of antenatal and neonatal
interventions). Healy made the distinction between science and engineering by reminding us, very bluntly,[9] that 'in contrast to the scientist, the
technologist is not concerned with truth at all.' 'The mark of the technologist is that he must act; everything he does has some sort of dead-
line. He has to manage, therefore, with as much truth as is available
to him, with the scientific theories current in his time; and if these are
subsequently proved to be untrue (the fate of all scientific theories), or
even known already to be so, he must still do the best he can.' Like
structural engineers, Healy notes, technologists are, in the best of
circumstances, influenced by the splendid institution known as factors
of safety: 'structural members are carefully designed to take the known
stresses according to the best available theories, and then are made
100 percent or so stronger again just in case the theories are not quite
right.' Not a bad operational model for antenatal/neonatal engineers
who are obliged to take well-meaning definitive action every day in a
world filled with uncertainty.

(1997)

In the early 1970s, there was a great deal of discussion among ethicists
about the possibility of cloning an adult human being; and they condemned research leading to this ultimate feat of bioengineering.[1] But
scientists rejected the criticism, claiming that critics created bizarre
scenarios; the frightening prattle, they charged, fuelled unfair suspicions
about the moral probity of researchers. Following this brief hubbub, the
topic of human cloning faded, to a large extent, from public consciousness; until 23 February 1997, when the world was jolted by an announce-
ment from Edinburgh. Embryologists at the Roslin Institute had
succeeded in creating a cloned lamb using DNA from an adult sheep's
mammary cell. Suddenly the ' bizarre scenario' returned as a topic for
impassioned debate!

The embryologist who carried out the experiments stressed that
the goal of the programme was the production of a wide variety of
pharmacological proteins (to be harvested in the milk of cloned sheep)
for the treatment of human ailments. 'We can't see a clinical reason to
copy a human being,' he said, '[and] we are briefing authorities to make
sure this technique is not misused.' But, as one medical ethicist pointed

out, 'The genie is out of the bottle, this technique is not, in principle, policeable.'

Unfortunately, the prognosis for social control of the new cloning technique, based on the history of the development of other powerful technologies, is gloomy. 'We have never limited a technology—or even approached limiting a technology—to its beneficial uses,' Kimbrell has pointed out (in comments about organ transplantation).[2] 'Society's past experience with both nuclear and petrochemical revolutions,' he observed, 'demonstrates that the more powerful a technology is at expropriating and controlling the forces of nature, the greater the disruption of our society and the potential destruction of life as we know it.' If the late Hans Jonas could hear about the amazing new potential for modifying human reproduction, he might be particularly alarmed. 'Granted that we can "take our own evolution in hand,"' he once wrote,[3] 'it will slip from that hand by the very impulse it has received from it: and here, more than anywhere else, the [old adage applies] we are free at the first step, but slaves at the second and all further ones.'

13

'... disavowing the tree'
(1990)

Life can only be understood backward, but it must be lived forward.

Søren Kierkegaard

More than 90 years ago, William Fletcher, a district surgeon stationed in Kuala Lumpur, conducted a controlled clinical trial[1] to demonstrate that a staple article in the Malaysian diet—white (Siamese) rice—was *not*, as claimed by some observers, the cause of beriberi. In a recent discussion of moral problems that arise in the conduct of such clinical exercises,[2] Vollrath examined Fletcher's critical experiment carried out during the second year of an epidemic of beriberi that began in 1905 at the Kuala Lumpur Lunatic Asylum. The asylum was considered to be an ideal location for the controlled trial, Vollrath notes, because the lunatics were a captive population whose living conditions could be altered at will.

The district surgeon, having obtained permission of the government to conduct the experiment, lined the residents up and numbered them in consecutive order; those with odd numbers were assigned to the east ward, even-numbered residents were sent to the west ward. Subsequent admissions were assigned to the two wards in alternate order. For one year, beginning on 5 December 1905, all the residents received identical rations except for the type of rice offered. The standard fare prior to the trial (which included Siamese white rice) was served in the east ward; residents in the (experimental) west ward received only Indian brown rice in the usual diet. Fletcher was surprised to find that his prior expectation (no difference in outcome) was not supported by the results. Beriberi occurred in 34 of 120 residents (18 of the affected died) on the ward receiving the standard (white rice) diet; among 123 fed the brown rice diet, there were no deaths and only two cases of beriberi (both of these residents were suffering from the disease when admitted to the asylum).

Just as Vollrath's account of the unexpected outcome in the old, almost forgotten trial in Kuala Lumpur was published, news of the abrupt termination of a modern large-scale controlled clinical trial with surprising interim results made headlines in American newspapers.[3] The present-day investigators were testing the efficacy of two drugs (flecainide and encainide—antiarrhythmia agents which slow conduction in cardiac tissue) accepted as proper treatment to suppress mild to moderate irregularities of cardiac rhythm (pp. 189–91). The drugs were in current use to treat more than 200 000 Americans with these conditions. In the formal Cardiac Arrhythmia Suppression Trial (CAST), outcomes were compared in enrolled patients who were allocated, in random order, to either an antiarrhythmia-treatment group or to a control group (the latter received 'dummy' pills). The trial, scheduled to continue through 1992, was stopped three years early when the safety monitoring committee overseeing the trial was convinced that mortality was unexpectedly higher (56 deaths) among 730 patients receiving specific-drug treatment as compared with 22 fatalities in the group of placebo-treated controls.

A comparison of the Kuala Lumpur and the American clinical trials provides supporting evidence for the claim that there has been considerable improvement in the safeguards to protect the rights of patients enrolled in such therapeutic experiments over the intervening period of more than nine decades. But we have found no easy answers to the many of questions discussed by Vollrath. Much of the difficulty he describes is related to a widespread failure to take into account the highly variable nature of evidence gathered at the bedside. There appears to be, for example, remarkably little appreciation of the interpretative difficulties that arise when relatively few patients become sick or die after exposure to some harmful influence (e.g. the majority of patients who ate white rice in Fletcher's experiment did *not* develop beriberi; the majority of the treated patients in the present-day cardiac arrhythmia suppression trial did *not* die).

The misunderstanding about variability leads to a poorly defined notion of a doctor's moral obligation to his/her patient in the conduct of clinical trials that test new therapies. As already noted above, one version of the profession's duty (termed the 'doctor's therapeutic obligation:' Always prescribe the best treatment) requires that doctors must not allow their patients to be enrolled in a controlled trial as soon as interim results show that a trend has developed in favour of one of the compared treatments.[4] But as pointed out, this view is as confused as that of a demented racing fan who demands that a horse race be stopped the moment one horse inches ahead of the pack to take the lead. Outcome of illness, like outcome at the track, is the result of a multitude of influences—the inescapable problems of interpretation related to variability cannot be solved without pre-planned stopping rules in the design of clinical trials (and in pre-agreement on the length of the course in a horse race!).

Results in both trials under discussion make the point that doctors need to recognise that they do have a 'study-design obligation' in the conduct of clinical trials. Patients' best interests are served when investigators take precautions needed in a trial format to improve the likelihood of making sense out of information. For example, a glimmering of the notion of 'study-design obligation' can be seen in Fletcher's conduct of the trial so many years ago in Kuala Lumpur. (Perhaps the action was related to the fact that he began the trial as a sceptic: 'at the commencement of the experiment the opinion was held by myself that rice was neither directly or indirectly the cause of beriberi.') Four months after the diet experiment was under way, Fletcher noticed that beriberi was occurring only in asylum residents receiving white rice. Acting on the possibility that brown rice might be protective, he began a crude crossover modification of the experiment: If a resident survived an initial attack of beriberi, the convalescent was transferred to the brown-rice ward. Ten such residents were transferred, all had no further symptoms. Since the admission of these patients caused some overcrowding in the brown-rice ward, four residents were transferred to the white-rice section of the asylum; two developed beriberi, one of whom died.

In the design of the recent antiarrhythmia trial, the inclusion of an untreated control group improved the chances of obtaining interpretable results; and, no small accomplishment (!), the concurrent control design reduced the number of patients exposed to the completely unexpected harmful consequences of the widely-used drugs. Like Fletcher's hopes for the standard white-rice diet, the present-day investigators expected that standard drug treatment would be vindicated by the trial results. (A small pilot trial conducted in 1982 had indicated that patients having problems with asymptomatic or moderate heart-beat irregularities might be protected from a subsequent heart attack or death by controlling irregular cardiac rhythm with antiarrhythmia drugs.) A member of the steering committee for the CAST trial said he 'was truly stunned and shocked' when given the interim results by the safety monitors.

Anyone can see, with the clear vision of hindsight, the safety and the fairness of the hedging strategy used in both trials: One-half of the enrolled patients were protected from the unfortunate consequences of what their doctors *did not know* about the treatments they prescribed. There must be increased public recognition that it is just this risk-limiting feature which makes concurrent control design a socially responsible exercise. (Medical positivists to the contrary notwithstanding, knowledge about treatment effects is *never* complete.) Moreover, for all enrolled patients in a comparative trial the unknown risks and hoped-for benefits are distributed impartially, as they are in everyday life, by chance. In response to reporters' questions about the practical value of the truncated CAST trial, one of the participating investigators said, 'Absolutely, unequivocally, this trial was a success because we have identified two drugs of a type that are more dangerous than the disease they are supposed to treat.'

Another issue stands out in an examination of the 1905–06 and the 1989 trials: the problem of who can, should, or must participate in these clinical exercises has not yet been solved. There has been some progress since the days of the Lunatic Asylum trial, insofar as there is general agreement that it is unconscionable to enrol institutionalised or mentally incompetent patients without obtaining explicit and informed consent from individual guardians. But the knotty problem of who is a proper enrolee is not completely solved by the now generally-accepted rule that only fully informed volunteers may participate. The informed-volunteers-only approach overlooks the dubious moral position of those who refuse. Do they have the right to insist, in effect, that others must undertake the risk on their (the refusers) behalf? What should we say about those who, as one critic has written,[5] are content 'to possess the end and yet not be responsible for the means, to grasp the fruit while disavowing the tree, to escape paying the cost until someone else has paid it irrevocably.' Chalmers has made a plea for an accounting of the public obligation:[6] 'we must face up to the fact that testing treatments is everyone's business.'

(1997)

There are no convincing answers to questions about fairness in the recruitment of patients in randomised trials. Volunteerism is widely accepted as the only ethical solution to the dilemma of who shall participate, because it honours the principle of respect for personal autonomy. But this interpretation of fairness is in conflict with the principle of social equity.

For the fairest possible distribution of unknown risks and hoped-for benefits, the precept of distributive justice would decree that every eligible patient must 'draw a lot.'[1] In time of war, for example, a national lottery is used to decide who, among all eligible young persons, shall risk their lives in battle. Here random sampling is accepted as a fair and democratic solution to the problem of extremely difficult choices. Interestingly enough, the case for equating participation in the battle against pain and suffering, with the civic duty of national service in conventional war, was made more than 50 years ago by Sigerist[2] 'The war against disease and for health,' he wrote, 'cannot be fought by physicians alone. It is a people's war in which the entire population must be mobilised permanently.'

There have been no calls for a mandatory lottery to ensure fairness in selecting participants for medicine's on-going war against disease. In fact, Hans Jonas, a respected moral philosopher, made a special point of denouncing conscription by lot for medical research, labelling a compulsory draft as 'threatening and Utopian'.[3] Although voluntary enrolment is accepted as impartial, this plan does not guarantee that burdens in the evaluation of new medical weaponry will be distributed equitably among all segments of society. We need to be attentive to the social status of enrolees and of 'refusers;' and we should record any social inequalities that result from voluntary participation in clinical trials.

14

Diffusing responsibility
(1990)

Responsibility is not a group concept. Sharing responsibility
widely is like having no responsibility at all.

F.A. Hayek[1]

In 1927, the story goes,[2] a secretary burst into her boss's office and
shouted, 'Mr. Smith! Lindbergh has just flown across the Atlantic all by
himself!' Smith, engrossed in reports, did not respond. She tried again,
'Mr. Smith, you don't understand—all by himself a man has flown the
Atlantic!' This time he looked up. 'All by himself a man can do anything,'
he said. 'When a committee flies the Atlantic, let me know.'

Anyone who has been forced to listen to endless drivel in pointless
committee meetings can understand Smith's disdain. But, Manchester
reminds us,[2] the age of soloists (Lindbergh was called the Lone Eagle) is
long gone. Like it or not, committees are here to stay. And the apocryphal
Mr. Smith underestimated the potential of group action (the camel, it is
rumoured, is a horse that was put together by a committee). We are
surrounded by evidence of the incredible accomplishments of committees: they created the atomic bomb, put a man on the moon, eradi-
cated smallpox ... transformed the world. We live in a superhuman
(some would say an inhuman) age fashioned by team players.

Clinical medicine, known in the past for its fiercely independent solo
players, has been transformed dramatically and, apparently, irrevocably
by group actors. A highly visible demonstration of new-age medicine in
action is provided by cardiopulmonary resuscitation teams, now a part
of the everyday scene in hospitals. Since the introduction of CPR, a little
more than 30 years ago, any and all patients seem to be candidates;
regardless of underlying condition, prognosis, and age. An editorial
writer has described the action:[3] the rescuers respond to 'crash' calls with
great enthusiasm and sprint to their destination; sending nurses, notes,
and screens flying along the way. Resuscitation hardware is deployed
immediately and the hyperactive team crowding around the patient's bed
begins the CPR routine with no lost motion. After rescue is well under
way, the team leader asks for details of the patient's diagnosis and recent

status. The assembled rescuers discover, all too often, that the patient has been steadily deteriorating as the result of an illness with a hopeless outlook. (Of 35 patients who underwent 36 CPRs in six months on the general ward of one hospital, there were only 2 long term survivors.[4])

Team players have also changed the scene in delivery rooms. Not so long ago, an extremely small or a badly malformed infant with poorly established initial breathing often was placed in a far corner of the room immediately after birth. The decision to withhold resuscitation usually was made by the obstetrician who knew the family, knew the parents' circumstances, and often knew the parents' wishes. There was little or no discussion of the dark drama by the few other attendants in the delivery room. Everyone tried to ignore the gasping respirations of the baby—death never came quickly enough to relieve their acute, but silent, discomfort. The outcome of delivery often was reported as 'stillborn.'

Beginning with the efforts of Virginia Apgar to focus attention on and to report the status of all newborn infants at age one-minute,[5] it became increasingly difficult to carry out the well-meaning deception. Moreover, as interest in marginal neonates increased, the number of caregivers in the delivery room rose, rescue routines were developed, team action was refined, and the numbers of babies reported as 'stillborn' decreased. Campbell recently recalled,[6] for example, that the incidence of stillborn infants with spina bifida fell in the early 1960s after the introduction of a more optimistic surgical approach to treatment. Note also that there is a steadily rising proportion of liveborn infants with low birthweight (under 1.5 kg) in England and Wales.[7] The most likely explanation advanced is that this trend is, to some extent, an artefact. Infants of gestational age less than 28 weeks, who in the past may have been classified as miscarriages and therefore not counted in birth registration, are now resuscitated and counted as livebirths.

It is interesting to reflect on the amazing change in attitudes and in action that have occurred when a marginal infant is born. Walker has reviewed the current situation:[8] with very few exceptions, those attending a delivery are obliged to resuscitate all infants born around 22–24 or more weeks of gestation. The delivery room is no place for 'snap judgements' about poor prognosis, Campbell argues,[6] particularly when the such decisions are made by relatively inexperienced young doctors. Walker points out[8] that a resuscitate-all policy provides the time needed to assess baby's status in some detail and to prepare parents for their loss before taking the irreversible step of allowing a marginal infant to die. He advises that doubts about viability and long-term prognosis should be discussed with parents. But there should be no mention of withdrawal of treatment, Walker stresses, until questions about such a move have been resolved sufficiently for the caregiving team to reach a decision among themselves. These arguments made to justify a policy of giving every infant a 'try at life' are reasonable, but where is the firm evidence that individual families and the community, are, in fact, best served by the aggressive approach?

It is, perhaps, a sign of how much we have changed since the days of the disdainful Mr. Smith that we have come to believe in the superiority of team-think: What we all agree to do must somehow be right, even when there are serious questions about acting on the completely unprecedented options made available by present-day antenatal/neonatal medicine. (In a slightly different context, Sass has raised[9] a central question about the dimensions of human responsibility in modern medicine; it is relevant to the resuscitate-or-let-be dilemma at the birth of an apneic or poorly breathing marginal baby. He asked, in essence: Are human beings obliged to keep their biological foundation intact, or must they manipulate the natural base?)

The sorry track record of action sanctioned by group agreement in the modern era should make us uneasy. For example, Freeman Dyson has tried to understand[10] how it came about that physicists (never known before, by any stretch of the imagination, to be team players!) were able to carry out the enormous collaborative effort that brought forth the first atomic bomb. The inconsistency put Dyson in mind of an incident that occurred in his childhood. When he was seven years old, he was reprimanded by his mother for an act of collective brutality in which he had been involved at school. A group of seven-year-olds, it seems, had been teasing and tormenting a six-year-old. 'It is always so,' Dyson's mother told him. 'You do things together that not one of you would think of doing alone.' This was a piece of his education he never forgot. 'Wherever one looks in the world of human organisation,' Dyson concluded, 'collective responsibility brings a lowering of moral standards.'

Reply by William B. Weil Jr.:

(1990)

As one who has for a long time been a member of groups (curriculum committees, nutrition committees, National Institutes of Health study sections, ethics committees, toxic substance task forces, etc.) I have experienced my share of the frustrations referred to above. I have witnessed group decisions that were mediocre and ones that were worse. Yet four attributes of the group process stand out. One was referred to by the commentator, two were not discussed and a fourth was given a negative value while I believe it has a positive one.

The one quality of group process that was discussed positively was the possibility of shared knowledge creating something that individuals alone could not develop. Although there are numerous examples in the industrial world, such as the space missions, and medical examples such as the eradication of smallpox, most of these represent application of ideas that were often the product of a single mind or of single minds building one upon another. Group activity on its own is unlikely to create a truly new idea.

The true values of group function lie elsewhere. One of these values is the mutual education of group members. Certainly it is my impression that I have gained more knowledge than I have imparted in the total of groups in which I participated. It is an exciting way to learn and a process that has found its way into contemporary medical education.

A second important set of values inherent in group activity is the opportunity to develop qualities of leadership and to hone one's capacity to dissent. Without good leadership and competent dissent, group productivity is rarely outstanding. Thus, individuals have an important role to play as individuals in a group and it is often in these roles that one may have the best opportunity to articulate one's values clearly. Many of us have been able to improve our understanding of our own values when required to express and defend them in the group arena.

But the question posed by Silverman regarding the group's value judgements requires a more specific response. It is my belief that the group value judgement can be more attuned to contemporary social mores than individual decisions.

When decisions are one individual's prerogative, there are about as many persons with poor moral positions as there are persons with high moral standards, and I would submit that physicians are unlikely to be an exception. As with trial by jury, it seems reasonable to assume that justice is more often served by a group than by one person's judgement. Individual decisions can run the gamut from egregious to excellent. Group process most often leads to regression toward some kind of societal mean. Unfortunately, while that protects society from the egregious it also tends to exclude the excellent.

Whether society in its totality, or as individuals, is better off with a narrower range of decisions or, in the long run, would be better with a greater range, accepting the bad with the good, remains a pertinent question. Certainly if all decisions made represented the mean, a tendency to mediocrity would seem inevitable. The editorial, 'The Golden Mean,' by Daniel Koshland Jr.,[1] makes this point very clear. But in the moral arena, where the life of an individual may be the issue, the capriciousness of individual decision-making (other than by the person directly involved or that person's duly appointed surrogate) seems a risk that is too great to accept. Thus, if my life were in the balance and I could not decide for myself and had not appointed a proxy of my own choosing, I would rather that an ethics committee decided the issue than having a random individual with that authority. What I would want for myself, I also want for others whether another adult or a newly-born infant. Let us not play Russian Roulette with human lives.

(W.A.S. - 1997)

The on-going debates about the resuscitate-or-let-be dilemma often fail to recognise the need for objective measures of the personal and societal costs of the vital decisions. The focus on moral principles in this controversy has overshadowed questions about the everyday consequences of the shift from the traditional approach (judgements based on a broad range of values, made by individual families and their personal doctor) to group decisions (a consensus based on a relatively narrow range of values, made by the caregiving team). Does a group-approved rescue policy (that ignores sharp individual differences in a family's social circumstances) in the high-minded effort to give every infant a 'try at life' increase or decrease the overall amount of pain and suffering and social chaos? Saving the lives of extremely small neonates in the first precarious moments and weeks of life requires enormous professional skill and prodigious resources. But these actions have proven to be very much easier to muster than the social operations needed to save such fetal infants from the miserable lives that await them in the chaotic, poverty-, crime- and drug-ridden circumstances in which so many must be reared—even in the richest and most highly developed countries.

15

Hawthorne effects
(1991)

Compliant patients have a remarkably intuitive ability to sense
what is wanted of them—and they provide it.

Anon

Do patients enrolled in randomised clinical trials receive better care, on
the whole, than others who receive the same treatments outside of the
context of formal study protocols? It is risky to make a judgement by
comparing outcomes in similarly-treated enrolled versus non-enrolled
patients because of selection bias (informed consent screens all candidates—only self-selected volunteers are enrolled[1]). Nevertheless, there is
a strong suspicion that an operational bias (the 'Hawthorne Effect') acts
to favour participants in formal therapeutic trials.

The research-setting-related phenomenon was recognised more
than sixty years ago in studies of the effects of different physical conditions on workers' productivity conducted at the Hawthorne Works of
the Western Electric Company in Chicago, Illinois.[2] During the years
1924–1927, the company's engineers, led by a representative from the
US National Research Council, set out to determine the effects of different
levels of illumination on workers' performance.

A series of experiments were mounted that gave confusing results. For
example, in one trial, women workers of equal experience in winding
induction coils on a wooden spool were divided into two groups: the
'test group' was exposed to successive increases in light intensity at set
intervals, and the changes were accompanied by appreciable increases
in production; but the 'control group,' with no change in lighting, also
increased production 'of almost identical magnitude.'

The puzzled experimenters then began to test the effects of decreasing
light intensity in graded steps: once again, production in both 'test' and
'control' groups increased slowly but steadily until the light level reached
three foot-candles. Up to this point, workers under 'test' conditions maintained production despite the discomfort and handicap of insufficient
illumination. Finally, two capable and willing workers were tested in a

locker room in which the light was reduced to 0.06 of a foot-candle (approximately equal to that on an ordinary moonlit night). Even under this very low intensity of light, the women maintained their work efficiency; they said that they suffered no eyestrain and that they tired less than when working under bright lights.

The surprising results led to a long series of experiments in the same setting at the Hawthorne factory over a six-year period (1927–1932).[3] A team of researchers from the Harvard Business School now sought to test the effects on productivity of changes in a number of working conditions. For predetermined periods, each of several weeks duration, the experimenters tried one and then another pattern of rest periods and refreshments, and also variations in the duration of the working day. Throughout each of eleven experimental periods, worker-output increased successively and substantially above prior levels. Finally, the researchers carried out a twelfth period of study in which conditions of work were returned to the original status: no specified rest periods, no refreshments, and a standard working day. For the twelve weeks of this final experimental period, daily and weekly output of each worker rose to a point higher than at any other time in the series of changes.

The unexpected steady upward trend in productivity, unrelated to any specific change in working conditions during the Hawthorne experiments, was not easily explained.[4] Interviews with the workers suggested that the mental attitude of the group of test workers had undergone a definite change during the protracted experimentation. The women felt they received special recognition as participants in the study and, as a consequence, were responding more to prestige gained than to any specified change in working conditions. These classic studies of the work output of Western Electric Company assembly workers established the Hawthorne Effect as a distinct and important influence in studies of industrial relations: 'The effect (usually positive or beneficial) of being under study upon the persons being studied; their knowledge of the study often influences their behaviour.'[5]

The non-specific Hawthorne Effect probably plays some role in determining outcomes in planned medical studies. Patients do tend to improve solely as the result of increased attentiveness on the part of caretakers. In parallel-comparison treatment trials, more attention is, in fact, given to the details of interventions than in everyday practice: enrolled patients receive increased personal notice, and the actions of caretakers, prescribed by study protocol, are closely monitored by overseers. It would be surprising if clinical trial participants did not respond favourably to the increased consideration; they are certainly aware of their special status as volunteers willing to undergo not-yet-fully-tested treatment, and they do gain social prestige.

It is probably useful to think of a study-related Hawthorne phenomenon in medicine as a summation of the familiar placebo effect related to patients' expectations plus subtle modifications in caretaking behaviour that comes about as a result of the expectations of investigators. The latter influences—they are classified as 'experimenters' effects'—have been tested extensively by social psychologists (see Rosenthal's famous Pygmalion experiment[6]). One of the strongest arguments for double-masking precautions in a comparative therapeutic trial is based on the hope that Hawthorne-like social influences will act evenly in both arms of the study when neither caretaker nor patient knows which of the alternative treatments under test has been given.

In all healer–patient encounters, particularly when there is uncertainty as to best treatment, there is a strong emotional interest in the force of action.[7] And there is evidence that a sizeable number of patients do understand that their participation in clinical trials is a positive action; that is to say, a decision taken in their own best self-interest. For example, a survey of the attitudes of current and potential patients (104 patients with cancer, 84 cardiac patients, and 107 members of the 'general public') revealed that a substantial majority of the respondents (210/295) believed that patients should serve as research subjects.[8] Asked why they might participate in clinical studies, a little more than half (152/295) selected the response 'to help me get the best medical care.' This optimistic response suggests that many patients regard their doctor's recommendation to participate in a clinical trial as equivalent to the doctor's best counsel with regard to treatment in the face of uncertainty. If these high expectations are at all typical, they place a heavy ethical burden on investigative clinicians.

Doctors are often told that they must not forget an old admonition,[9] 'You should treat as many patients as possible with new drugs, while they still have the power to heal.' The caveat needs to be kept in mind when projecting the optimistic conclusions reached at the end of even the most carefully designed and rigorously executed randomised clinical trial. It is not too surprising that trial results do not always translate well into everyday practice—particularly when practitioners and their patients are not fired up with all of the ritual, faith and enthusiasm that characterised the formal study.

Even though present-day treatment is more powerful and certainly more specific than ever before, the amazing power of suggestion in investigative settings is worth remembering. For instance, 12 patients with long-standing itching skin eruptions were enrolled in a study ostensibly to test the effectiveness of four orally administered antipruritic agents.[10] Four envelopes (each coloured differently and marked A, B, C, and D) were given to each patient with instructions to take tablet A four times a day for two weeks, followed by tablet B four times each day for two weeks, and so on, until tablets in all four envelopes were consumed over a period of eight weeks. Eight of the twelve patients reported improvement with one or more of the preparations; three patients were helped by tablets in all four envelopes; one patient reported that tablets A and B made her 'jumpy and nervous,' another said C and D made her feel 'groggy.' All the tablets were identical lactose-containing placebos.

'You easily believe,' the Roman poet Terence noted long ago, 'what you hope for earnestly.'

(1997)

Another fascinating demonstration of the 'Terence phenomenon' associated with study enrolment has been reported recently in the treatment of benign prostatic hypertrophy.[1] A Canadian trial conducted by urologists in 28 centres, compared the effects of finasteride versus a placebo (flour pills) for a two-year period in the treatment of 613 affected men. Shrinking of the prostate (by more than 21%, on average) and improved urine flow were observed in men allotted to the finasteride-treated group. On the other hand, men in the placebo-treated group also experienced improved urine flow, even though their prostates had grown, on average, by over 8%. And some of the latter patients continued to do very well: 'Some didn't want to stop taking the [flour] pills,' said the author.

A professor of preventive medicine found the prostate study results 'remarkable.' '[The placebo] did not really change the direction of the disease,' he said, 'it just changed one of the indicators.' A similar experience was reported many years ago in a small double-blind trial of internal-mammary-artery ligation for angina pectoris.[2] The degree of improvement was judged to be greater in controls (who received a sham operation) than in patients whose vessels were ligated! The surgeons reported that, 'One patient, who had been unable to work because of his heart disease, was almost immediately rehabilitated and was able to return to his former occupation. He reported a 100 per cent improvement at six months and 75 per cent improvement after a year. His arteries were not ligated.'

16

Power plays

(1991)

Of all tyrannies, a tyranny sincerely exercised for the good of its victims may be the most oppressive.... [T]hose who torment us for our own good will torment us without end for they do so with the approval of their own conscience.

J. Lewis[1]

The name 'John Doe' had its origin in English Law: a fictitious name for a party, real or hypothetical, to any transaction, action or proceeding. In recent years, the surname, in a diminutive form as 'Baby Doe', has acquired a new life and a surprising new connotation in America. The term to provide a sheltering anonymity was used first in a judicial action in the United States to protect the privacy of a specific family and one neonate; soon the anonym was used in the news media and in everyday speech to refer to the class of infants born with life-threatening biological impairments.

The infant who came to be known as 'Baby Doe' was born on April 9, 1982 in Bloomington, Indiana.[2] The baby was afflicted with Down's syndrome complicated by oesophageal atresia and tracheo-oesophageal fistula. When the parents refused to allow surgical intervention, the hospital sought a court order to compel corrective treatment. A judicial hearing was convened at the hospital on the following morning; the baby's condition and prognosis were described and conflicting opinions were put forward. Some doctors advised immediate corrective surgery, others recommended that no active treatment be attempted. The father testified that after conferring with the experts, he had signed a statement authorising the passive clinical management set out by the doctors who were not in favour of surgery. The judge ruled in favour of the parents: 'Mr. and Mrs. Doe, after having been informed of the opinions of two sets of physicians, have the right to choose a medically recommended course of treatment for their child in the present circumstances.'[3] The hospital appealed the decision to the Indiana Supreme Court where the parents' refusal to allow surgical intervention was upheld without a written opinion and the record of the case was ordered sealed. The infant died at 6 days of age.

There was wide publicity about the events in Bloomington, and about similar unhappy situations that soon turned up. Before long demands were heard for government action to prevent what was seen by then-President Reagan, by right-to-life groups and by advocacy organisations for the handicapped as unfair discrimination against children with disabling conditions. The clamour led directly to a series of regulations designed to require life-preserving treatment for extremely premature infants and others with severe impairments. The new rulings, issued by the Department of Health and Human Services,[4,5] came to be known as the 'Baby Doe Regulations.'

The bureaucratic actions ushered in a short-lived, but nonetheless very bizarre period in the history of American paediatrics. Providers of health care services to infants were required to post a notice in prominent places, declaring that 'Discriminatory failure to feed and care for handicapped infants in this facility is prohibited by federal law [the US Rehabilitation Act of 1973];' a 'Baby Doe Hotline' telephone system was set up to receive anonymous reports of instances of non-treatment; and 'Baby Doe Squads' were readied to conduct on-the-spot investigations of all allegations of discriminatory non-treatment. The rules for the outlandish witch hunt were soon declared invalid in a federal court[6] on the grounds that they were 'arbitrary and capricious,' but the court hinted that 'some regulation of the provision of some types of medical care to handicapped newborns' might be needed.

The controversial issues were far from settled in the minds of protagonists; the matter continued to receive wide news coverage and there were bitter debates whenever the families of other 'Babies Doe' refused corrective treatment for life-limiting defects. Further rules were issued and these were struck down on grounds that the Rehabilitation Act was never intended by Congress to apply to medical decisions about newborns. Finally, in what was seen as compromise legislation, the US Congress in 1984 passed amendments to the Child Abuse and Neglect Prevention and Treatment Act.[7,8] The amendments defined the withholding of 'medically indicated' treatment from an infant as a form of child abuse and neglect, rather than as an act of discrimination. Now (in what has become known as 'Baby Doe Regulations II,' but are, in fact, guidelines to define medical neglect) it is widely perceived by doctors that the federal law requires 'treatment (including appropriate nutrition, hydration and medication) which in the treating physician's . . . reasonable medical judgement, will be most likely to be effective in ameliorating or correcting all such (life threatening) conditions.'[9] This life-preserving treatment, according to the guidelines, can be withheld only when infants are in an irreversible coma, or dying, or when such treatment would be 'virtually futile' and its provision would be 'inhumane.' The guidelines reject a future-quality-of-life standard as a criterion for providing life-preserving treatment to a severely impaired neonate.

The new regulations required only that individual States of the Union, if they wish to receive federal child-abuse protective service grant funds, must have programmes that respond to reports of medical neglect (as defined in the guidelines). Most doctors concluded, however, that there was now a new legal standard for medical action. As a result, the privacy originally intended with use of the term 'Baby Doe' is a sham under the interpretation of the new American rules. Parents of affected infants have, in effect, lost their rights to make 'active treatment vs passive care' decisions in the privacy of their home based on the counsel of family members, loving friends, and trusted religious and medical advisers. The momentous decisions that will determine the well-being over the full life-time of every family member are now made in the hospital—an unreal theatre-like setting in which the actors are doctors, ethicists, and, not infrequently, judges. Often these decision-making authorities are strangers—they have had little or no past contact with the family. Although a trend toward limiting parental autonomy began years before the tumultuous events of 1982–84, American families have experienced an abrupt loss of power as a direct result of the every-day interpretation of the new legislation.

The blinkered demands of Baby Doe Regulations II have ignored the social, cultural and spiritual diversity that has guided decision-making in the practice of medicine throughout history. Moreover, the outlook of the guidelines is certainly not shared by all people in contemporary society. As noted above repeatedly, many view unlimited neonatal treatment as unreasoning; heroics often conflict with the parents' and the community's interpretation of what constitutes social responsibility.

A poll of American neonatologists suggests that the new rules are responsible for a change in the standards of care in that country.[10] Most (81% of 494 respondents) disagreed with the statement that Baby Doe Regulations II would have the effect of improving care for all infants. Two thirds (66%) disagreed with the statement that the regulations did not affect parental rights to consent or refuse treatment based on what is in the infant's best interest. About half (56%) the respondents agreed that most critically infants are now overtreated when the chances for their survival are very poor. A poll of the opinions of affected families has not been conducted.

The shift of power in the United States from decision by parents and trusted advisers to decision in accordance with a government decree about what constitutes medical neglect should alarm parents and doctors in all countries. The experience brings to mind a warning attributed to C.S. Lewis'. 'Man's power over Nature,' he noted, 'is really the power of some men over other men, with Nature as their instrument.'

(1997)

The overiding concern of bioethics for 'personal autonomy'—protection of patients' from arbitrary acts of paternalistic doctors or reckless researchers—has been tempered, in recent years, by recognition that this frame is much too confined (pp. 193–95). For example, as Murray has pointed out,[1] 'Wherever the powerful seek to impose their will on the powerless, autonomy, along with justice, should be our battle cry. But autonomy can only be a part of the story about how we are to live together, how we make families and communities that support the growth of love, enduring loyalties, and compassion.' Nelson has also argued against a narrow focus on the rights of 'splendidly isolated individuals.'[2] We should, he urged, 'design a system of medical decision-making sensitive to a broader range of values.'

A group of American parents, whose children had serious neonatal medical problems, has now come to the same conclusion. They have published a set of 'Principles for Family-centered Neonatal Care'[3] in which they declare that doctors 'must recognise the life-long impact of their treatment decisions on patients and patients' families.' 'We reject the notion,' the parents assert, 'that our children are well-served by laws mandating life-sustaining treatment without regard to pain and the quality of life.' As critically-ill newborn infants cannot say 'no' to extreme medical interventions, the Family-centered Principles affirm, 'parents must have the right to refuse excessively painful, burdensome, or unproven therapies on behalf of their infants.' These forthright-declarations by families may help to restore a sensible balance of decision-making power in American neonatal units, after years of confusion brought on by the unfortunate Baby Doe brouhahas.

17
Unbridled enthusiasm
(1991)

A tale is told of a man in Paris during the upheaval in 1848, who saw a friend marching after a crowd toward the barricades. Warning him that these could not be held against the troops, that he had better keep away, and asking why he followed these people, he received the reply, 'I must follow them. I am their leader.'

A. Lawrence Lowell (1856–1943)

The bitter memory of the thalidomide incident more than thirty years ago and the grave lesson taught by that tragedy have, for the most part, faded from public consciousness.[1] It is important to remember, however, that a loud public outcry at the time was directly responsible for American legislative action (the Kefauver-Harris Amendments to the US Food, Drug and Cosmetic Act in 1962) which spelled out unprecedented requirements for proof of safety and efficacy in well-controlled clinical trials before a new drug is released for general use.[2] Now vociferous objections to these restrictions are voiced by patients with acquired immunodeficiency syndrome (AIDS). The loud demand for deregulation has alarmed those who remember the past. They fear a return to the time of uninhibited therapeutic exuberance—days that were interrupted, periodically, by explosive iatrogenic disasters (particularly in neonatal/perinatal medicine).

The current turn of events reminds us that we cannot obtain highly reliable evidence about a new treatment without the full co-operation of relatively large numbers of suffering human beings. What happens when the sufferers, desperate for miraculous cures and in no mood to hear that magical treatments are rare, refuse to listen to warnings about the possibility of disastrous consequences that may follow a quick incautious introduction of new treatments?

The question has surfaced in the experience with what is called a 'parallel track' to test proposed drugs. The plan is in use for the first time as part of the clinical evaluation of dideoxyinosine (DDI) for the treatment of AIDS.[3] Preliminary tests suggested that despite serious side-reactions the new agent did have an anti-viral effect which warranted a formal comparison with zidovudine (AZT), the established standard treatment. While the conventional controlled trial of DDI vs AZT is under way, DDI is also made available, on a 'parallel track' to patients who are not eligible or who are unwilling to enrol in the formal exercise. As it turns out, so many patients have elected to receive DDI the researchers despair of enrolling enough patients to complete the randomised trial.[3] According to one rough estimate, almost 20 times as many AIDS patients have signed up for uncontrolled use of the untested drug than have joined the comparative trial.[4]

One researcher has noted that the 'parallel track . . . is an invitation to disaster. . . it will prevent us from finding drugs that will help people.' Another pointed out that 'DDI is a toxic drug and the only way to know if its benefits outweigh its risks is to assess it in clinical trials with large numbers of people that compare it to the standard treatment.' It was also recalled that if formal evaluation with concurrent controls had not been carried out before it was released, 'AZT would have been completely dismissed as a drug that's too toxic.'

A spokesman for AIDS patients points out that *all* of the affected are desperate for treatment of their fatal illness.[5] Early release without concurrent controls (also called 'expanded access' and 'compassionate release') makes DDI available to many with no other options for treatment (those who are not eligible for the randomised trial, those who live too far away from trial sites, patients who have been unable to tolerate standard AZT therapy). AIDS patients contend, with understandable impatience, 'Any program that has the potential to save lives deserves a chance.'

The patients are absolutely right when they argue that concurrent controls are unnecessary when evaluating new treatment of disorders with a very high mortality. Historical controls provide a reliable contrast if, and it is a very big IF, the arguments are confined to the category of uniformly fatal conditions. Unfortunately, real-life situations are rarely this simple. It has been noted,[6] very accurately, that patients with severe and fatal disease represent only the 'tip of an iceberg.' There are almost always many more patients with milder forms of the same disorder, and increased interest in case finding takes place when a promising new treatment is introduced. This leads, invariably, to the recognition and treatment of less severely affected patients. As a consequence, outcome in currently treated patients appears improved over past experience, even when the treatment is without effect or is, it turns out not infrequently, harmful.

Many people are thoroughly convinced (and the popular view is bolstered by the frequent and enthusiastic accounts of medical 'miracles') that a truly effective new treatment produces a clear-cut difference in outcome and that improvement is easily documented by a simple head-count in a series of consecutively-treated patients. But such immediately obvious 'slam bang' effects (like the effect of penicillin in syphilis) are quite rare. The modest beneficial effects and the harmful complications of today's powerful innovations are extremely hard to recognise without rigorously-designed trials.[7]

The history of a surgical procedure (porto-systemic vascular shunt in hepatic cirrhosis) provides an instructive example of the inverse relation-ship that is often seen between the rigour of clinical study design and doctors' enthusiasm for the new treatment under test.[8] The operation, introduced in 1945, was reviewed 20 years later: in 65 reports of results, enthusiastic support for the treatment came from groups who conducted uncontrolled or poorly controlled studies; in the majority of well-controlled studies, there was either no conclusion or doctors reported little or no enthusiasm for the procedure as an effective measure to improve survival. Similar examples of an inverted association between quality of clinical evidence and doctors' enthusiasm for specific inter-ventions have been reported in the field of cancer research.[9]

It would be extremely cruel to discourage AIDS sufferers by dwelling on the difficulties in interpreting uncontrolled clinical studies, and by reminding them that the search for effective treatment is slowed by reli-ance on these weak and often misleading exercises. But the leaders in the battle against AIDS who are now following the crowd marching along the 'parallel track' approach to new treatment should not delude them-selves. They would do well to keep one of Hugo Muench's most enduring aphorisms in mind:[10] 'Nothing improves the *apparent* performance of an innovation so much, as the lack of controls.'

(1997)

Despite heightened awareness of the need for organised scepticism about all claims made in clinical medicine, it would be foolish to ignore the yearning of all sufferers for magic and certainty. It is remarkable how many sensible patients can be hoodwinked by the overblown claims for implausible therapies like imagery, spiritual healing, megavitamin therapy, energy healing, massage, and a colourful variety of empirical folk remedies.

For example, a national survey in the US found that the number of visits to unorthodox healers was greater than the total number of calls made in 1990 to all primary care medical doctors nationwide.[1] An editorialist explained,[2] 'the reason people go to nonmedical practitioners is simple: they want to feel better. Access is easy. Invitations to be healed are everywhere. It's cheaper than seeing a physician.... [and] Anecdotes and testimonials from friends are powerful persuaders.' Oliver Wendell

Holmes (1809–1894) recognised the flight of reason that occurs when our lives or well-being are threatened. Over 100 years ago he wrote:[3]

> There is nothing people will not do, there is nothing they have not done, to recover their health and save their lives. They have submitted to be half drowned in water, half cooked with gasses, to be buried up to their chins in the earth, to be seared with hot irons like slaves, to be crimped with knives, like codfish, to have needles thrust into their flesh, and bonfires kindled on their skin, to swallow all sorts of abominations, and to pay for all of this, as if to be singed and scaled were a costly privilege, as if blisters were a blessing and leeches were a luxury.

18
Caring and curing
(1991)

All my means are sane, my motive and my object are mad.
Captain Ahab, in *Moby Dick*

The spectacular success in the treatment of infectious disease and other ancient life-threatening disorders with 'miracle drugs' in the years immediately after the Second World War provided a solid base for soaring optimism about future medical victories over all human illness. Medicine seemed to be, at last, on the threshold of the millennial age envisioned three centuries earlier, at the very beginning of the scientific revolution. For example, in 1655, a prophetic outlook of the 'most noble' goal of medicine was expressed by Samuel Hartlib, a physician:[1]

> I would have you understand my Prognostication of the true universal medicine. There grows in Paradice a Tree, which is called the Tree of Life....and in the glorious and long expected Coming, the fruits of it shall be gathered, by which all men shall be delivered from death... And this glory and great joy hath God reserved for Us that live in these latter days, and hath kept his good Wine until now, I do foretell another Garden will be found whence shall be had herbs, that shall preserve men not only from sickness, but from death itself.

Many death-defying 'herbs' have, indeed, been found in the past few decades and, so it has appeared to many enthusiasts, we seem to be well on our way to the paradise of physical perfection and immortality forecast by Hartlib. But sober realists are not easily convinced. Rene Dubos has warned about 'the mirage of health.'[2] 'Complete and lasting freedom from disease,' he wrote, 'is but a dream remembered from imaginings of a Garden of Eden.' Moreover, in the past few years, the enormous cost of an endless series of miracle treatments has given rise to some doubts. Can we, the sceptics are now asking, afford miracle medicine's full cost, involving, as it does, the enormous outlay of community resources and many disturbing long-term social consequences?

It is not surprising that doubts have turned up in the United States, since it has committed a larger share of its national treasure to health care than any other country—with no discernible superiority in health status of its citizens. (Health expenditure in the US rose from 5.2 per cent of the gross domestic product in 1960 to 11.1 percent in 1986; in the UK, the corresponding outlays were 3.9 per cent in 1960, increasing to 6.2 per cent in 1986.)[3]

The current financial crisis with respect to medical care in the US is widely perceived to be related to the means of delivering services: a wasteful and unfair non-system for rendering medical care simply cannot cope with the explosion of demands and of costs which have come with rapid technological development in medicine. According to the conventional wisdom, if there was sufficient political will, a cost-effective and equitable national health care plan could be enacted to provide every American with medical care according to individual need. Now a vigorous and fundamental dissent from this orthodox view has been put forward by an American medical ethicist, Daniel Callahan,[4] director of The Hastings Center in New York. The underlying difficulty is not with economic or moral means, he proposes, but with the chosen ends. The goals and the ideals of present-day medicine and health care have not been closely examined, nor have they been seriously challenged.

Like the 800 pound gorilla who sits wherever he chooses, the problem of resource allocation generated by limitless medical progress is now overpowering. 'The very nature of medical progress,' Callahan argues, 'is to pull to itself many more resources than should rationally be spent on it, often more than can be of genuine benefit to many individuals, and much, much more than can be socially justifiable for the common good.'

The current American view sees health as a boundless good and an end in its own right; it allows individuals the freedom, indeed the right, to define their own health needs; and it allows individuals to demand, in the name of the health privilege, the help of fellow citizens to meet those self-defined needs. Americans begin, Callahan notes, by asking what individuals need for good health; the community's concerns are subordinate. He wants to reverse the priority: 'How much and what kind of health do we need for the common good, and what will collectively and communally help and improve us as a society?'

Respect for individual needs and dignity must not be ignored, but these requirements should be placed in social perspective. Callahan argues that persistent emphasis on individual need has left the US with the impossible task of solving the social problem of allocation: How should collective resources (with ingredients that are private and individual) be distributed? We will never get all the health care we think we need as individuals (particularly with widely varying definitions of the need in a plural society like the US). He points out, 'We have lost our way because we have defined our unlimited hopes to transcend our mortality as our needs, and we have created a medical enterprise that engineers the transformation.'

Callahan makes a strong plea for the primacy of caring over curing: 'There is never any certainty that our illnesses can be cured or death averted, eventually they will, and must triumph.' The plea is timely because of the steady increase in chronic illness. The glamour of cure in modern medical 'warfare' tends to overshadow the universal need to relieve the pain and suffering of the incurably sick and dying. Callahan recognises that the vulnerability to sickness and death can only be reduced, never vanquished. (Life is a universally fatal, sexually transmitted disease.[5])

The arguments for assigning a relatively less important place to expenditure for spectacular never-say-die medical treatment, while increasing funds to improve the social circumstances in which illness occurs (education, housing, poverty, public safety, ...) are not likely to endear Daniel Callahan to medical positivists. But he is not alone in questioning the national priorities. For example, more than 20-years ago, when neonatal intensive care was beginning to expand dramatically in the US, Professor Laura Nader, a sociologist at the University of California, asked some probing questions about the newly visible activity:[6] '[W]ho benefits, ... the companies that produce the life-support machinery, the doctors who work at this labor, insurance companies, the hospital, the parents, the families of the newborn infant, the baby? How has our society come to be spending so much time and money on neonatal intensive care,' she wanted to know, 'without similar attention to born-healthy but later not-so-healthy, deprived children?'

The pertinent questions remain unanswered and neonatal intensive care in the US has expanded enormously—the cost is now estimated to be at least US$2.4 billion per annum.[7] Recently, Leon Eisenberg, Professor of Social Medicine at Harvard, also called attention to the grossly unfair apportionment of effort and of resources,[8] 'Our nation has done superbly well in neonatal intensive care...yet, the melancholy fact is that the United States is 20th in the world in overall infant mortality...[and] the reason for the failure is not obscure.' Mortality rate for black infants is twice as high as that for whites and there are similar differentials within the white population: the highest rates are found among those on the lowest rungs of the socio-economic ladder.

(1997)

The above-noted 'unfair apportionment of effort and of resources' in the US has been acknowledged recently by a politician—Richard Lamm, the former Governor of the State of Colorado.[1] He agreed that there is a preoccupation with ethical issues concerning individual autonomy, yet the dubious ethics of the overall health care system is completely ignored. 'We myopically obsess about individual trees,' he observed, 'while the whole forest is being clear cut.'

Lamm cited instance after instance in Colorado of excess capacity of hospital beds, high-tech diagnostic machinery, heart surgeons, neonatologists... all sitting 'cheek-by-jowl with great need.' And he cited a telling example of the obsession with individual cases while overlooking the injustice of the delivery system for health care. The story began when Oregon made an effort to distribute care more equitably in that State by stopping payment for organ transplants, until all people below the poverty line were provided with basic health care. When one patient died after he was denied a transplant, the resulting outcry was 'volcanic'; the unhappy incident made the front page in all of America's newspapers. 'Yet it is instructive to compare what California did when confronted with a similar choice,' Lamm pointed out. The California legislature voted to pay for transplants; then, 'one week later they knocked 270 000 low-income Californians off the Medicaid rolls. California killed far more people than Oregon did—but Oregon got all the criticism.'

The ex-Governor made a strong plea for fairness. 'We must recognize,' he opined, 'that the ultimate ethical question is not how to give all the "beneficial" medicine to each individual, but how to maximize the health of the community.'

19

On the edge
(1992)

Man's special gift is reason, as a bird's is flight. His highest calling, then, is to overcome his biological instinct to breed in great numbers and to extend his range of habitation—to use reason, to do the one thing no other animal can do, that is to limit himself voluntarily.

Edward Austin Abbey (1852–1911)

In his Croonian Lecture of 1988,[1] Professor David Hull noted that scientific interest in the possibility of sustaining the life of a marginally viable newborn infant by 'artificial means' goes back at least three centuries. He quoted minutes of a Royal Society meeting on 27 January 1663:

> Dr Merret acquainted the Society that he had received information from Naples, concerning a person, who had an art of keeping newborn infants alive without respiration, for a good while. It was thought very desirable to have further enquiry made into the matter, both as to the truth of fact, and the way of performing it, viz. whether it was done by hindering the closure of the foramen ovale, which is supposed to shut soon after the birth of the animal.
>
> Mr Croune suggested an experiment of keeping a new cast puppy in warm milk to see how long it would live without air. He was desired to be curator of this experiment....[Dr Croone, as he was later addressed, was the first Registrar of the Royal Society and as such was usually required to perform the experiments]

The interest of Royal Society appeared to be purely academic; no mention was made that knowledge acquired by the warm-milk experiment might have some immediate practical application in the care of non-breathing human infants. In point of fact, the extremely high mortality rate soon after birth (the 'expected loss' in all animal species, including our own throughout all of human history) was not, until about 100 years ago, perceived to be a problem requiring systematic remedial action.

Concerted medical intervention to keep all human offspring alive began in France during the last quarter of the 19th century. Thomas Cone, the

American paediatric historian, notes[2] that the tremendous loss of life as the result of military action and famine during the Franco-Prussian War (1870–1871) had left the French nation quite discouraged. By 1880, the size of the wartime losses seemed even more ominous because the annual birth rate in Germany was then twice the rate in France. One doctor speculated that if the inequality continued, 'in forty years Germany would be able to put under arms a total number of conscripts double the number available in France.'

The French infant welfare movement which began in the 1870s, Cone observes, was motivated by concern that deaths would exceed births: 'It was primarily the declining birth rate that led to an intensive investigation of the causes of the excessive infant mortality and means of prevention.' A Commission on Depopulation was deputised to make this study and to put forward recommendations that would remedy the alarming situation. The investigations led to the establishment of a number of innovative programs; as a result, France became the pioneering leader in the development of an organised infrastructure for maternity and infant welfare.

Two patriotic obstetricians in Paris, Stéphane Tarnier (1828–1897) and Pierre Budin (1846–1907) extended the national rescue efforts to include the large number of 'congenital weaklings' (principally prematurely-born babies). They organised an effective system which provided favourable 'artificial conditions' (convectively-ventilated closed incubators and expert nursing care, especially gavage feedings) for the survival of the 'weaklings.'

The French example of organised action to rescue marginally viable neonates was taken up only haltingly in other countries. For example, the birth rate in England and Wales fell from 34.7 per 1000 in 1871 to 28.5 in 1901. In 1902, J.W. Ballantyne pointed out,[3] 'the steady fall in the birth-rate in the British Isles as well as in some foreign countries and in our own colonies, has... caused an appreciation in the value, economic as well as sentimental, of the premature infant.' He stressed the urgency to conserve the lives of these marginal babies: 'It may not be possible exactly to define their value to the state and the community, it is greater now [in 1902] than it was when the birth-rate was 35 per 1000 [in 1870].' Despite this plea, nearly thirty years elapsed before the first British organised program for premature infant care was established in Birmingham.[4]

In the United States at the turn of the century, there was little interest in preserving the lives of marginal infants. Cone quotes the observations of one observer in 1900, '... [of] the thousands of premature infants born in the United States annually....most are quietly laid away... little if any effort [is] made for their rescue. It is only in the home of the childless or where offspring were greatly desired that any considerable efforts were made to save them.'

As pointed out previously, the early reluctance to mount substantial campaigns to preserve the lives of 'weaklings' was based on widespread doubts on the part of doctors. For instance, in 1900, one American physician noted[5] that many of the families of the feeble infants lived in appalling social conditions: 'these infants had come from wretched tenements, and, as the result of exposure, ignorance and neglect, had been nearly moribund when received at the hospital.' Another probably spoke for others in the community when he asked,[6] whether 'these small lives justify all this trouble to save them.' Many parents also had a fatalistic outlook and saw the death of their weak baby as an expression of God's will. In the present era, doctors and parents still have mixed attitudes about the advisability of making intensive efforts to prolong the lives of all infants by 'artificial means' without taking into account social consequences.

Feverish scientific investigation in the past few decades has brought about a vastly improved understanding about the pathological mechanisms which account for the wide variety of disorders responsible for the high risk of death in the neonatal period. And highly effective 'artificial means' are now available to keep alive many severely compromised newborn patients. As a result, the disparity between the intensive care provided for infant rescue and the social circumstances of the family in which a child will be reared is, in too many instances, greater than at any time in the past.

To take an outrageous hypothetical example, it would be possible to fly a well trained and fully equipped neonatal intensive care team to a famine-ridden country in Africa to save the life of a severely compromised neonate using the most advanced 'artificial means' of life support. Who would even consider a project with such bizzarely mangled priorities for medical care? And yet fragile neonates are rescued every day in developed countries, when it is clear to all the rescuers that their skilfully executed intricate medical action is a prescription for social disaster in the immediately foreseeable future.

An American pioneering neonatologist, Mildred Stahlman, has asked (in connection with newly proposed treatments for medical complications in premature infants):[7] 'Is treatment enough?' She noted that premature birth often occurs in connection with such severe social problems that the medical condition of mother and infant are of secondary importance. 'It is to the socially disadvantaged of our country—the poor, the unemployed, welfare recipients, the undereducated, school dropouts, the medically underserved, teenage mothers (frequently, unloved children), the poorly fed, the inadequately housed, all those for whom the stress of day-to-day living and survival is of paramount importance—that the majority of premature infants are born.'

In addition to troubling questions about the full social consequences of heroic rescue, there are many unanswered medical questions, still, about the exact 'artificial means' to prolong the lives of infants born at the edge of viability (under 28 weeks of gestation). Hull predicts that 'trying harder with the current approach which has been effective in more mature infants is probably not going to be good enough; we are likely to go on as we are, saving some after a frightening struggle and losing others.' 'With this predictable outcome,' he advises, 'parents must be given an option of making another infant.'

(1997)

There are still many questions about the fairness of using all-out measures for rescue. All too often the lives of the 'saved' neonates are exposed (after discharge from the hospital) to life-endangering risks comparable to those found in Third World countries. The pietistic declarations of love and concern for the welfare of children are hypocritical, because, as noted above, so many extremely fragile infants are reared under horrendous conditions in the gritty ghettos of major cities.

Quinn recently described[1] a familiar scenario on the obstetric ward in the hospital of a major American city: 'a 15-year old mother was giving birth to her second baby; her first child having been born two years earlier. While she was in labor, her boyfriend, the reputed father of the new infant, sat in the delivery room and sucked his thumb. The grandmother, a young woman herself, was too drunk to stay awake during the delivery.' But highly skilled rescue teams regularly ignore these ominous signs of future disaster, when, for example, they make decisions to initiate all-out technical means to give every seriously malformed or marginally-viable neonate 'a chance at life.' No one seems to ask the question about long-term responsibility when the 'chances' are so poor: Who should be held accountable for the predictable increase in the level of social chaos in the community that results directly from this high-minded, but short-sighted, rescue-all outlook?

John Rawls, the American philosopher, spoke out about the issue of accountability[2] in a discussion of the principle of 'procedural justice.' He pointed to familiar directions on how to divide a cake fairly: 'We simply require the person who cuts the cake to have the last piece.' When applied to decisions about rescuing marginally-viable neonates, justice dictates that if no competent parent is available to raise the infant, that responsibility should fall on the shoulders of the rescuer. Interestingly, a form of Rawlsian accountability does appear to guide action in China, where the cost of high-tech neonatal medicine is very high. Renzong reports[3] that 'if the physician insists on treating an infant with serious birth defects, the parents say, "Yes, if you pay the cost." However,' he explains, 'the income of the physician is roughly the same as the parents—in the [US]$40–50 per month range.'

20
Informing and consenting
(1992)

I think informed consent is a farce...The information [given parents] is what I want it to be.

An American neonatologist

Until fairly recently, patients who appeared on the doctor's doorstep were seen as self-directed supplicants. The sick arrived, seemingly, as the result of their own free will. Many patients expressed their need in the form of a plea: 'Please do everything possible, Doctor!' For countless ages, healers interpreted such voluntary submission as clear evidence of unrestricted consent for any and all treatments, including untried experimental interventions. Practitioners responded with enthusiasm and with imagination.

The requirement of formal and specific consent for a medical action, particularly the notion of patients' *informed* consent for previously unevaluated treatment and for medical exploration to improve understanding, is a relatively recent development.[1] The new stipulation has been put in place to restrict the time-honoured paternalistic predilections of the medical profession. The beginning of a change in prevailing attitudes can be traced to a startling incident that took place in America in 1963[2]—the appalling episode called attention to the need for critical examination of long-standing informal arrangements for the conduct of bedside research.

The incident began when a young resident physician at a chronic disease hospital in New York was approached by the director of the department of medicine who asked whether the houseman would be interested in participating in a clinical project conducted by two experienced and highly regarded cancer researchers. The study, funded by the US Public Health Service and already under way at two other institutions, involved the subcutaneous injection of live cancer cells in order to measure the rate of rejection of the foreign cells by weak, debilitated, chronically ill patients. The rate was to be compared with the findings after similar injections already given to cancer patients in a famous American cancer institute and to healthy 'volunteers' in a state prison.

In July 1963, each of twenty-two patients in the chronic disease hospital received a test injection—it was completely unrelated to their usual care. The helpless patients were not told they had been selected by the houseman to be participants in a clinical experiment. The soon-to-be-infamous episode precipitated stormy debates among the hospital's doctors and these led to investigations by the hospital's grievance committee and by the board of directors. One member of the hospital board took the hospital to court to force disclosure of the hospital records—soon details of the incredible cancer-cell experiment foisted upon unknowing, feeble patients were broadcast world-wide by the media of mass communication.

The public clamour following revelation of the cancer-cell-injection affair and subsequent charges by Beecher,[3] an American anaesthesiologist, concerning 'unethical clinical studies' (many were carried out on prisoners, soldiers and the mentally retarded) led to governmental action in the form of a memorandum by the US Surgeon-General.[4] The directive, dated February 8, 1966 and entitled 'Clinical Investigations Using Human Subjects,' was sent to the heads of institutions conducting research with Public Health Service grants. For the first time, clinical investigators supported by federal moneys were required to obtain prior review of studies involving patients by a human investigation committee convened in each institution. The critical pre-examination was to include 'the appropriateness of methods to secure informed consent.'

The effect in the US was immediate and dramatic: informed consent suddenly became a highly visible step in the planning of all clinical studies. Although questions about unwarranted hazards to patients had not been uncovered in treatment trials using randomised-control design, the impact was felt immediately in this form of clinical investigation. Consent procedures were now reviewed prospectively and they became a central concern in the design of human trials.

All investigators were not convinced that this well-intentioned fiat was needed or that it would, in fact, protect patients against abuses by experimenters. In the 1960s, controlled clinical trials were being conducted with increasing frequency and conviction following the path-finding British streptomycin trial reported in 1948.[5] Prior to the arrival of formal consent in 1966, many clinical investigators were quite convinced it was disingenuous to claim that all patients or their surrogates could be made to understand the technical details at issue in comparative treatment trials. It was cruel many felt, to frighten patients by asking them to share the burden of the treating doctor's uncertainty revealed by a consent ritual in therapeutic trials.

Sir Austin Bradford Hill recently reviewed the climate of opinion at the time of the influential 1948 trial, when formal patient's consent was not deemed an ethical requirement. Reflecting on the change that has occurred since that time, he saw the need for an ethical committee to oversee the *doctors* during the planning and the conduct of a clinical trial. He noted, however, 'I think it is wrong to shift the entire consent-giving responsibility onto the shoulders of patients who cannot really be informed or know what weight *relatively* to put upon the technical information provided concerning risks and benefits. The doctors, it seems to me, must weigh all this in the light of their medical training. It is my personal opinion,' Sir Austin concluded, 'that the responsibility rests with them and their sense of morality.'

From the very outset in the informed consent era, which is now more than two decades old, there have been doubts of the kind voiced by Sir Austin. Is it ever possible to determine whether trial participants, or their surrogates, have been fully informed? Is the signature on a consent-form a reliable indicator that an enrolee has given true consent? Has *pro forma* informed consent succeeded in providing more protection for enrolled patients than in the pre-1966 era? Although there have been endless pronouncements and opinions, it has been discouraging to see so few experimental studies to determine outcomes after various formats of the consent ritual.[7]

There is a strong suspicion that the consent formality introduces volunteer bias[8] and functions as an unjust social filter. For example, Harth and Thong[9] examined the sociodemographic characteristics of parents in Australia who volunteered their children for a randomised trial of a new drug for asthma. When compared with parents who refused, volunteering parents were found to be less well educated, fewer had professional or administrative jobs, they had less social support, they exhibited greater health seeking behaviour, and they consumed more habit forming substances. The Australian findings support a gnawing concern that well-meaning efforts to prevent cavalier actions of research doctors have not solved the knotty problem of assuring that the burdens of participation in clinical research are distributed justly. If the Australian experience is at all typical, children enrolled in clinical trials are likely to come from families that are more socially disadvantaged and more emotionally vulnerable than are the families of children whose parents refuse to grant informed consent for enrolment in a comparison trial.

The endless squabbling about informed consent will not end until some way is found to explore discretionary formats that will balance the concerns of patients, their families, doctors, legal experts, bioethicists, and the community at large. So long as the loud arguments remain so heavily burdened with opinion and so weakly challenged with concrete evidence, the outlook for progress seems very dim indeed.

Reply by William B. Weil Jr.:

(1992)

As indicated above, the process of informed consent has been extensively discussed in the medical and ethical literature, but it has had very little critical study. The plea that it is time for the scientific community to undertake such investigations can be enthusiastically endorsed.

This writer's concern arises from another aspect of the commentary. If the unproved efficacy of the informed consent process were to lead to its abandonment until effectiveness is established, that would be a disservice to medicine and to society. The reason for considering such a possibility is that this is what may happen in other areas of medical intervention. When a medical professional considers a treatment or procedure that has not yet been determined to be efficacious, it is often prudent to suspend the utilisation of such treatments until definitive, carefully controlled studies have demonstrated whether the treatment is useful or not. I would urge that we not adopt the same attitude toward the practice of obtaining informed consent, even though the effect of the informed consent procedure on the well-being of patients, and on the credibility of research studies which involve informed consent, has yet to be delineated. To forego this procedure until its efficacy is, or is not, established, would be unfortunate.

Informed consent is a term used to describe a process which derives from the concept of personal autonomy. Personal autonomy has a variety of dimensions or components, but ultimately reflects a principle of human behaviour which holds that a competent individual should have the right to determine those discretionary risks he/she is willing to accept for whatever benefits he/she perceives may result. This principle of behaviour rests on the more fundamental attributes of personal liberty and privacy.

As the author of the above commentary indicates, the concept of personal autonomy has only recently been applied to medical care and research. Until the past few decades, personal autonomy in medicine was limited to the decision to seek medical care, and even that discretionary act was, and still is, not always available as an option. Nevertheless, once an individual has sought medical care, the decisions involved in such care were made by the physician, a practice termed paternalistic. Personal autonomy, in contrast to paternalism, is now generally accepted to apply rather uniformly to participation in medical research.

There is somewhat less agreement about the application of personal autonomy in the use of 'innovative therapy,' i.e. treatment which is not yet firmly established as beneficial, but which in the mind of the physician is likely to be more helpful than harmful. Still more controversial is the acceptance of personal autonomy in the provision of 'routine,' or well-established, medical care.[1] It is also recognised that personal autonomy, which professed to be one's governing doctrine, can be easily contravened operationally by the nature and the extent of disclosure of risks, benefits and alternatives that is actually practised.

Informed consent, whether written out briefly or in great detail, given verbally, or even implied, is designed to be the formal expression of the nature of the interaction between the patient and the physician, investigator, or other health care person. The actual form in which the informed consent is expressed is often a legal, procedural or personal issue which, while important, is not the basic concern. The fundamental question is whether the interaction between the individual patient and the health care provider is based on the principle of personal autonomy or paternalism.

The basic question raised by Silverman can be rephrased: Has the institution of the informed consent process actually altered the provider/patient interaction in the direction of increased personal autonomy and decreased paternalism? This question is one that, at least in theory, should be able to be empirically investigated, and such investigation ought to be done.

In the view of this writer, the process of informed consent should continue to be endorsed, however, even if the answer to the previously mentioned question was negative at the present time. The premises on which this view is based are:

1. Personal autonomy in medical decision-making is an appropriate goal.

2. Changing human behaviour may be a complex and time-consuming process which is only partially understood when applied to large groups of individuals such as the population of physicians.[2] Nevertheless, it is possible, ultimately, to change behaviours, even those of physicians.

The first premise is based on a personal value system; the second deserves some further elucidation.

At least three factors seem to play a role in generating changes in group behaviour: knowledge, incentive and reinforcement. The continued use of the informed consent process contributes to each of these factors. By requiring an expression of informed consent for medical research involving human subjects, and by encouraging its use in innovative and routine medical care, increasing numbers of patients, physicians, investigators and other care providers will become acquainted with the procedure, and ultimately will understand the more fundamental basis (increasing patient autonomy) which the procedure is designed to reflect. Thus, knowledge will be enhanced.

Increasing use of the process of informed consent will gradually generate a social norm which then becomes an incentive for others to behave in a similar fashion. As such behaviour becomes more wide-spread, its repetitive use, when accompanied by underlying changes in attitudes, should increase patient satisfaction and ultimately improve society's perceived valuing of the medical profession. As this social change occurs, the result will reinforce the providers' behaviour and the cause of personal autonomy will have been well served.

Intentionally, the application of these issues to the use of surrogates making decisions for children and incompetent adults has been omitted. While the underlying principles are equally applicable to children and incompetent adults, such individuals may be compromised by their in-completely developed cognitive capacity to express their own personal autonomy. Furthermore, it is semantically not possible to provide informed consent for another person if one cannot know that person's own views. (This does not necessarily apply to previously competent adults who may have expressed their own views when competent.) For children and permanently incompetent adults, the term informed permission by a surrogate, with or without the personal affirmation of the subject, may be the more appropriate constructs for reflecting similar values in these individuals.[3]

(W.A.S. - 1997)

Although it has been argued that informed consent obtained in clinical research should be the same as the consent obtained for routine medical care, the ideal is not easily achieved. There are stubborn differences in the extent of disclosures made, and in the candour of doctors, in the two situations.[1] When obtaining consent for participation in a randomised trial, doctors are required to reveal the justification for the study. As a consequence, they are obliged to reveal that there is not enough evidence to support a rational, informed choice for one of the two or more treatments under investigation. On the other hand, when doctors ask for consent to use an intervention in ordinary care, they minimise all uncertainties about the 'best' treatment on offer. Physicians feel duty-bound to provide patients with an unequivocal, confident recommendation for action.

Additionally, a difference is rooted in the legal ground rules. In research settings (as noted earlier), investigators are *compelled* by regulation to obtain informed consent in words set down and approved in advance by an ethics committee. In everyday practice, doctors are merely *exhorted* to solicit consent by an appeal to medical ethics or to legal self-interest, and the words used in the consent ritual are reviewed, if at all, only in retrospect.

A group of Australian oncologists have now urged[2] correction of the imbalance between the consent required in randomised trials and in routine care, by requiring identical rules and formats in both situations. Additionally, they advise, all refusals-to-enrol in trials should be formally documented. In an 'informed refusal' form, patients should acknowledge that they are voluntarily forfeiting the protection afforded by the rando-misation plan approved by the institution's ethics committee. Only this hedging strategy can guarantee that the chances for a hoped-for benefit and the risks of unpredicted harm of the treatment on trial are to be distributed in the safest way that can be devised—by lot.

21

Lifesavers
(1992)

Medicine is the [profession] most likely to attract people with
high personal anxieties about dying.

S.B. Nuland[1]

Thought is the prisoner of language, and thoughtful action is influenced
heavily by the choice of words. For example, physicians often conjure
up rescue fantasies and talk of 'saving lives' when they employ heroic
measures to prolong the lives of patients who are deathly ill. The doctors
understand, of course, that the time and the place of a rescued person's
demise have merely been changed by an act of medical heroism. It is
impossible to 'save a life,' as an evangelist 'saves a soul,' for an eternity.
Earthly existence can only be prolonged for varying finite periods.
We pay a certain price for using the 'save-a-life' metaphor when this
mental-set guides medical interventions.

In the adventurous new field of neonatal medicine, onlookers are
often puzzled when they hear doctors talk about 'saving' seriously compromised babies by aggressive interventions. For example, a journalist
and a hospital chaplain have written a very perceptive account[2] of
the attitudes and behaviours of caretakers observed in a prestigious
American special care baby unit over a period of 18 months. They found
that the young doctors (neonatal medicine is a young person's game) who
endured the exhausting physical and emotional demands of complicated
high-tech treatments, seemed to view the intensive care nursery as a war
zone—an arena where special forces and armaments were deployed
against death and disability. Interns and other trainees spoke of being
'on the front lines' or 'in the trenches'. As in other highly demanding,
dangerous enterprises, the protagonists found it necessary to develop
smooth working teams. Doctors and nurses came to know one another
well, the reporters observed, 'they help one another in crises, they hold
together against the rest of the world, knowing that nobody who has
not shared their experience can fully understand. They develop their
own special ways of seeing and doing things, their own special language

and humour. In effect,' the observers concluded, 'they become a separate small society... with its [own] unique culture.'

A professor of political science became interested in the new phenomenon of rescuing previously doomed neonates born extremely early or with serious biological imperfections. He arranged to spend four months observing the social structure, the outlook, and the technical operations of personnel in an American neonatal unit. He wrote,[3]

> This place is like a magnet to me. I can't pull myself away. Why? Because it is like going in the best magic room at a state fair with all the latest lights and equipment and magicians performing fantastic tricks with the highest-priced prizes at stake—health [and] life....

He observed that the hardworking young staff was coping, as competent persons tend to do in tense situations, by joking to stay relaxed and to reduce the unrelenting pressures of life-and-death decision-making. After answering a phone call to the nursery, a doctor shouted, 'MASH unit! Incoming wounded!' The team members seemed to be supremely confident of their technical power to 'save lives.' In an interview, a resident said, '[we] can bring a peach back from the dead, with the skills [we] have developed.' (In another setting,[4] a nurse asked an intern, 'Who gets saved?' '[A]lmost anything,' was the reply, 'We'd resuscitate a Big Mac if we could.') When initiating heroic action in a life-threatening emergency, the medical team often took the position that parents were too distraught to make rational decisions about interventions for their babies. The political scientist concluded that the special care nursery was 'a place where decent and dedicated people do and think terrible things.... [T]he conditions of the place make them what they are, whatever they are.'

Two sociologists conducted a field enquiry by 'entering the life' of an American newborn intensive care unit for a period of six months; and, over an eight-month period, they followed a consecutive series of seriously-ill babies admitted to the facility.[5] They also found a preoccupation with 'saving the lives' of compromised neonates. The director noted,

> We have made a real difference here, not just in mortality rates in the city, but over an entire region, even into [an adjoining state in the US]. There are infants who wouldn't be alive now if we hadn't started this unit.

The neonatal team ascribed the highest importance to 'technological truths:' in hospital care, 'technology was the sole pragmatic means to the end of curing.' The approach inspired the belief that technology 'fosters a progressive, rational order.'

What stands out in the reports of these and other interested (non-medical) bystanders is their amazement to find that dedicated, intense young doctors seemed to view every death of a marginal baby as a personal failure. Next time, the dauntless young 'warriors' seemed to say: next time, with a little more knowledge, a little more technical ingenuity, a little more effort, we will be successful in overcoming death—the enemy.

How *do* doctors come to hold such narrowly-focused death-defying views? Why *is* proficient action so much more highly prized than inactive reflection? The questions interested a group of health educators;[6] they postulated that the degree of activism in treating neonates with severe defects might be related to the level of development of a young doctor's moral reasoning. (The thesis was based on the work of Kohlberg[7] and Rest:[8] 'the differences among people in the ways they construe and evaluate complex moral problems are determined largely by their concepts of fairness, ... more adequate and complex concepts of fairness develop from less adequate simple ones.' Individual moral judgement matures and becomes less arbitrary, Kohlberg and Rest argue, with an increase in the amount and in the complexity of social experience.) From the results of a survey of American paediatricians, the health educators concluded that doctors whose moral reasoning is relatively high (e.g. mature consideration is given to a balance of interests) can be expected to be sensitive to characteristics of each situation and to vary their treatment accordingly (e.g. to be less aggressive in their treatment of neonatal defects in instances where the family requests such limits). 'Low [relatively immature] moral reasoners seem to treat cases more uniformly,' the survey team found.

John Emery points out that a 'never-say-die' attitude is seen more often among paediatricians than in other medical specialities.[9] 'Paediatrics is probably the speciality that is least concerned with death,' he writes, 'and to some extent is the anti-death phase of medicine.' The veteran paediatric pathologist notes that paediatricians become so closely involved with patients and their families that 'When a child dies [in an intensive care unit, the young] doctor is often emotionally exhausted.' Emery pleads 'that paediatricians need considerably more help in dealing with themselves' [when children under their care die] than they or most of their colleagues realise.'

Perhaps there would be some improvement in the way neonatal paediatricians cope with their 'defeats', if they would give some thought to a change in the language used to describe their 'victories.' Instead of talking about 'number of lives saved,' the young warriors might adopt the phrase, 'number of lives prolonged' to describe their miraculous results. The word 'prolonged' does not slip off a doctor's tongue quite as familiarly as the word 'saved'; and the suggested terminology does not have the connotation of completeness or of finality. But that is just the point!

Clergymen, it should be noted, choose their words carefully when they discuss the notion of *saving* a life. For example, Lord Soper once said, 'It is ludicrous that people who confess to the most ardent desire to get to heaven, use the most scrupulous precautions to keep themselves here on earth. What right has any of us to prevent anybody from beginning his journey home?'

(1997)

As Nuland, a perceptive surgeon, has noticed,[1] many doctors are attracted to a career in medicine because of their own heightened anxieties about dying. Given the vaunted image of doctors' God-like power over life and death, the lure is not too surprising. For example, the rescuer's personal stake in staving off death was revealed in an interview of a famous anaesthesiologist.[2] She told the reporter that she always carried a small surgical knife and a length of tubing in her purse to create an artificial airway in an emergency. 'Sixteen times I used it—successfully,' she said. 'Nobody, but nobody, is going to stop breathing on me.'

The predilection of doctors, even early in their training, to see the battle against death in personal terms, was bared in a dramatic episode played out on an emergency ward some years ago. A medical student had just started to examine a very old, unconscious man newly admitted to the ward, when the patient stopped breathing. The student called for help, a CPR team responded, resuscitative efforts were initiated quickly and extensively, all to no avail. The team left, leaving the budding doctor alone with the dead patient. The student was so disturbed by this unexpected disaster he lost all self-control, and began to beat on the dead man's chest while shouting, 'Goddamn it, you can't do this to me!'

22

Belief and disbelief
(1993)

Lack of belief is an act of faith; the one thing we can be sure of
is uncertainty.

John Mortimer[1]

Two decades ago, Eliot Freidson, a distinguished American sociologist,
wrote a very thoughtful book[2] in which he traced the historical development of society's notion of a 'profession' (an autonomous form of labour,
one which 'has gained control over determination of the substance of its
own work'). He used the occupation, which came to be called 'doctor of
medicine' as a revealing example of the evolution of idea and of action.

Firstly, Freidson argued, there is an important difference between
occupations that he labelled the 'consulting' professions, as distinct from
types of work that are usually referred to as the scholarly, learned or
scientific professions. The former are expected to solve the practical
problems brought to them by ordinary people; the practitioners can
survive only if they earn the confidence of a demanding clientele by
providing what are perceived to be effective problem-solving services.
The learned professions are expected to be the 'repositories and elab-
orators of theory and imputed knowledge;' to prosper, they need only
gain the interest and the patronage of a powerful sponsor—there is no
need to secure the confidence of the public at large.

The two types of occupation may be assigned to a single general class,
an 'autonomous profession.' However, the conditions for the establishment and maintenance of the two subclasses are so different, it has been
pointed out,[3] they should be considered quite separately. For example,
medicine first attained the status of a learned profession in the Middle
Ages, Freidson notes, with the rise of the university in Europe and with
the heightened importance accorded higher learning by the elite. The
university-trained doctors gained the support of the state and they
became the arbiters of medical work. However, medicine did not become
a truly 'consulting' profession (and control over its own work did not become fully operative) until the work itself became desirable and attractive

to the general public. The latter development took place a little over one-hundred years ago, after the construction of an increasingly solid scientific foundation (particularly after discovery of the bacterial cause of disease). Only then did the work of medicine begin to be generally recognised as superior to that of folk practitioners and other self-professed 'healers'. Prior to the relatively recent historical developments, the university-trained physicians were unable to establish a monopoly over the work of healing, Freidson concluded, because they could not create widespread public confidence and extensive use of the certified physicians' services.

There has been, of course, an incredible explosion of scientific information in very recent times, and medical practice is now increasingly dependent on the greatly expanded body of knowledge. Nonetheless, when sufferers consult physicians, the usual plea is, still, a very old one: 'Doctor, do something—anything!' As a result, the practitioner is under strong social pressure to adopt a different point of view about his/her work, as compared with the outlook of the academic investigator. 'The assumption by the public that the expert [practitioner] is competent, creates a sort of pragmatic compulsion,' Larson has pointed out,[4] 'to certify his worth in the eyes of the laity, he [the practitioner] must act.' Although, effective action is, certainly, highly desirable, action with very little chance of success is preferred over watchful waiting. Talcott Parsons has labelled this gambler's-fallacy-like attitude an 'optimistic bias;'[5] it turns up in 'situations wherein there is an important uncertainty factor and strong emotional interests in the force of action.'

Needless to say, the practitioner is very likely to be convinced about the utility of what she/he is doing; to believe, as Freidson emphasized, that what is done does more good than harm, and that intervention makes a difference between success and failure, rather than no difference at all. The belief-in-action model of therapeutic behaviour provides a clue to why it is so hard to convince doctors that the untested interventions they believe in, however strongly, must be formally evaluated prospectively.

The problem of insufficient participation in clinical trials (because clinicians are reluctant to enrol their patients) has been examined in some detail recently by Deber and Thompson of Toronto.[6] In an ingenious three-stage survey of Canadian physicians, concerning the proper treatment of breast cancer, the researchers found that favourable attitudes to the principle of randomized clinical trials were attenuated when doctors did not believe in the treatment regimens under test in a specified hypothetical trial. They also found a lack of consensus about the appropriate treatment for breast cancer (the disagreement was labelled 'macro-uncertainty'), and the collective doubt was matched with the high-confidence of individual physicians in their own treatment decisions (this strong belief was termed 'micro-certainty'). It seems, the researchers concluded, that in precisely those clinical situations generating the greatest controversy, and in which comparative trials are most necessary, are the very situations in which it is most difficult to obtain doctors' co-operative participation.

The 'individual-certainty / collective-uncertainty' syndrome, described in Canada, is certainly not an isolated phenomenon. The paradoxical situation is encountered over and over again whenever plans are made to mount randomised clinical trials to test controversial innovations. But, as Deber and Thompson emphasize, the strong beliefs of individual clinicians should not be ignored, if there is to be any hope that the results obtained in formal trials will influence subsequent medical practice. Attention to the factors that practitioners identify as important to their treatment decisions, the Canadians advise, should improve 'the extent to which clinicians believe that [trial] results can be extrapolated to individual patients.'

We cannot be reminded enough, it seems, that faith in personal clinical experience is not the same as faith in God. The important distinction between strong belief systems in medicine and in religion, lies in the fact that only the former are susceptible to disproof.

(1997)

What can account for the 'maxi-uncertainty: mini-certainty' paradox observed (above) in the treatment decisions of Canadian practitioners? Ann Lennarson Greer, an American sociologist, has been intrigued by these puzzling behaviours that indicate a disjunction between research evidence and everyday medical practice. An explanation can be found, she proposes,[1] in the social dynamics of two distinct cultures in the profession of medicine.

Like Freidson, she points out that the academic investigator and the bedside practitioner arrive at their callings through different routes of socialisation and indoctrination. 'For both groups a principle problem, perhaps the principle problem, is uncertainty,' she emphasises, 'but the approaches taken to resolve a state of doubt are different. Medical scientists turn to the design of formal tests to control for confounding variables in efforts to distinguish between rival hypotheses. On the other hand,' she notes, 'clinicians generally proceed inductively; they are preoccupied with the puzzles of individual cases, and with generating *experience-based post hoc* hypotheses. The practitioner's calling demands closure, and uncertainty is resolved through action: diagnosis and treatment. Science is abstract and open-ended,' Greer asserts, 'practice is concrete and forces closure.'

In interviews of over 400 community-based doctors, Greer, found that they developed 'numerous means of wresting action from uncertainty:

repeating what has worked well enough before, following the actions of role models, and conforming to the practice standards of local colleagues.' And the front-line doctors were often so suspicious of the motives of academic experts, there was little meaningful communication between the two cultures—as in the above-noted Canadian paradox. '[U]niversity researchers get so wrapped up in ideas they have pioneered, it becomes impossible for them to be objective,' one practitioner declared. Another cautioned: 'Research is like motherhood; there is no such thing as an ugly baby.'

23

Preferences
(1993)

One man's meat is another man's poison.

Lucretius (94?–55 BC)

The civil rights movement against social injustice in America, led by blacks during the 1960s and '70s, was contagious. It was followed by similar revolts against the status quo in other parts of the world. Many groups (ethnic minorities, students, women, gays, the disabled...) who experienced social alienation and feelings of powerlessness were emboldened to demand an active role in decisions affecting their lives. Patients' discontent about medical power also began to surface during this period (notably in the battle of women for control of their own bodies[1]). The struggle has persisted to the present day (for example, the anger of parents about unauthorised aggressive treatment of their extremely premature or malformed neonates pp. 23–25). At a time when the war against disease is chalking up more victories than at any time in history, patients are demanding participation in the decisions about how and when to exercise the awesome 'fire' power. Medical warfare is too important, critics are saying, to leave to the medical warriors.

The growing difficulties are revealed in the questions raised about how doctors decide to treat individual patients. As medical interventions increase in number, in complexity, and in cost, an individual doctor's decisions will almost certainly be monitored and challenged as never before. The sharp break with doctors' traditional 'clinical freedom' is described in a discerning series of articles by Eddy.[2] He reviews approaches taken to formulate policies for guiding decisions in clinical practice, and he points out the need to develop guidelines that are responsive to the hopes and desires of individual patients. The time has come, it seems, to challenge a Procrustean model for decision making. (Procrustes, according to Greek legend, was a robber who placed all his victims upon an iron bed. If they were longer than the bed, he cut off the overhanging parts; if shorter, he stretched them until they fit the prescribed size.)

Eddy suggests that an 'invisible hand,' as in Adam Smith's 18th century model of the marketplace, has determined medical practice policies in the past. The policies have rarely been designed and adopted according to a formal plan. By tradition, they have come about as the result of a continuous tracking of practices in general use. The 'invisible hand,' operating through individual decisions, has been counted on to ensure that correct ideas survived, that wrong notions were discarded, and that 'the collective medical consciousness [would] slowly... converge on the correct policy.' Appropriate practices were determined by the collective actions of practitioners, whose actions were themselves guided by the policies. The traditional approach used circular reasoning to advise that 'everyone should do what everyone is doing.'

The free-competition-of-ideas approach is being replaced slowly by organised efforts to set policy. It is important, Eddy points out, to examine the methodological rigour used in these formal exercises as a guide to the content of the directives. He distinguishes four approaches:

1. 'global subjective judgement' (there are no explicit analyses of relevant issues, the opinions of policymakers are presented, *ex cathedra*, in the form of a consensus statement);

2. an evidence-based approach (consciously anchors a policy, not to current practices or beliefs of experts, but to experimental evidence);

3. an outcomes-approach (not only anchored to available evidence, but explicit estimates are made of the magnitudes of outcomes associated with alternative practices); and

4. a preferences-based approach (a full description of evidence that includes magnitudes of all outcomes of interest to patients, and assessments are made of patients' preferences for these outcomes).

The wide variation in 'standard medical practice' from one locale to another has provided a very good clue that something is amiss: a critical examination of practice-policy issues is long overdue. For example, in the 1970s, Wennberg noted[3] marked geographic variations in treatment of benign prostatic hyperplasia in the United States (in one community, ten per cent of men over 85 years of age with BPH underwent prostatectomy; in other locales, the proportion treated surgically was as high as fifty per cent). He and his co-workers set out to examine the differences in doctors' practice styles that might account for the striking disparities. Beginning in the 1980s,[4] they invited leading physicians in the state of Maine to join in an on-going examination of the puzzling findings. The BPH study has turned out to be an instructive model for evaluations of clinical decision-making—Wennberg has coined the term 'outcomes research' for this kind of investigation.

Discussions with practitioners and a review of the evidence extant revealed an unresolved conflict about the indications for prostatectomy.

Some held that the procedure should be performed early as a preventive measure; others argued that watchful waiting was justified because the need for surgery was not inevitable, life expectancy was not extended, and many patients were content to live with their symptoms. The BPH study team found (from published reports, insurance claims data, and interviews before and after prostatectomy) that surgery was, in fact, associated with reduced symptoms and with improved quality of life for most patients. But this outcome was seen only in the men who were willing to accept the risks of surgery (these included death, failure to improve symptoms, impotence, and incontinence). Wennberg and his co-workers found that the decision to undergo prostatectomy depended, to a considerable extent, on patients' preferences for outcomes and their attitudes toward risk. No objective criteria (from history, physical examination, or severity of symptoms) were found that were accurate predictors of the preferences of individual patients for surgery or for watchful waiting. 'The subjective factors of risk aversion and personal tolerance for disease symptoms thus emerge,' they concluded, 'as important elements of rational choice.'

'If doctors choose differently,' the investigators argued, 'so can their patients.' The enlightened insight led to the development of a program ('Shared Medical Decision Making Procedure') to provide patients with the quantitative information—the probabilities for outcomes after available treatments in appropriate prognostic subgroups—as a first step in helping them make an informed choice. The investigators found that probability estimates for some outcomes important to patients were not available. It was clear that these estimates must be obtained by prospective investigation, but what study design should be used to obtain the missing probabilities?

When doctors must make a choice of treatments, they have come to rely on the power of experimental design in randomised clinical trials to provide estimates of the relative size of the principal effects of medical interest (difference in mortality or morbidity between compared treatments). But it is not clear that RCT results (in volunteers who consent to treatment allotted by chance) provide the reliable estimates needed for situations in which decisions are made by patient's choice.[5] Under the proposed rules for shared decisions, Wennberg's group is exploring a prospective observational study called a 'preference trial:'[3] 'the systematic follow up of patient cohorts where treatment assignments are made according to informed patient choice rather than by randomisation.'

The proposal acknowledges doctors' limited ability to determine what treatments and what outcomes patients value most. In place of the rigid 'Procrustean model,' a flexible 'restaurant model' for decision making is envisaged. Doctors provide continuously updated estimates of probabilities of all outcomes of interest for each of the treatments on the 'menu.' Each patient is free to make a choice based on the objective information provided plus uniquely personal considerations of the kind that influence all private decisions affecting life and well being.

Although nonexperimental studies provide relatively weak evidence about causation (a presumption that any observed difference in outcome is caused by difference in treatment), the goal of 'preference trials' is descriptive (a noncomparative estimate of the outcome to be expected after choice of an available treatment). Moreover, Wennberg's group is attempting to learn how to help patients make decisions consistent with their preferences. The free-to-choose approach recognises that the way in which people actually cope with decisional conflicts in their lives is quite complex.[6] Additionally, the explorations should provide testable assumptions about the advantages and limitations of basing treatments in prospective clinical trials on patient preference rather than on randomisation.

The current interest in preference-based studies is a healthy development (notice that a study design which takes clinician preference into account has now been proposed[7]). It should also be noted that distraught parents of seriously comprised neonates have long recognised the need to develop flexible shared-decision rules—sensitive procedures that take full account of families' preferences. Extremely difficult questions about treatments continue to turn up in the practice of antenatal and neonatal medicine. With any luck 'outcomes research' might become an idea whose time has finally come to the delivery room and to the special care baby unit.

(1997)

When examining the topic of parents' preferences for treatment of their newborn offspring, a distinction needs to be made between 'preference studies' (surveys of parents to determine the acceptability of proposed interventions) and 'preference trials' (assessment of consequences when a prospective cohort of parents make real-life choices of proposed treatments for their trial-eligible infants). Additionally, as Till and co-workers advise,[1] preference studies should be viewed as supplemental, not as alternatives, to randomised trials. A comparison of the outcomes of selected treatments with any other experience is always questionable, because there is no assurance that potential confounders (both known and unknown) will be distributed in the compared groups strictly in accordance with the laws of chance.

On the other hand, a comparison between randomised and non-randomised groups may, on occasion, reveal information that would otherwise be missed. For example, Henshaw and others[2] examined the relationship between pregnant women's preferences and the acceptability of two methods for first-trimester abortion (medical induction versus vacuum aspiration). Almost half of the women (168 of 363) expressed a preference; the remainder (195 of 363) were willing to undergo either method, and these undecided women were randomly allocated to one of the alternatives under test. Follow-up questionnaires revealed no important difference in acceptability among women who had expressed a preference (they were treated by the method of their choice). Among women with no expressed preference (the randomised group) there was a difference in satisfaction with treatment given. Most of the women allocated to receive vacuum aspiration were satisfied; only two indicated they would opt, in future, for a different method of abortion. But 21 of the women assigned to the medical regimen said they would choose another method next time. Without a patient-preference arm in this study, the authors concluded, the difference in approval would not have been unearthed.

A distinction needs to be drawn[3] between informed choice (in which patients or surrogates rely on estimates of the size of risk and benefits of proposed treatments) and subjective preference (in which patients choose to ignore the available evidence, and prefer to rely on prayer, on a hunch, or the advice of friends, relatives, or seers). While there is wide agreement that the RCT is the only reliable way to compare therapies, there is no clear view of how best to proceed when randomisation is either impossible or unacceptable to most patients. Perhaps ongoing studies will help decipher the complex interaction between doctors and their patients when faced with the need to act under conditions of uncertainty.

The most difficult hurdles to overcome in these situations are related to the widespread misconceptions about the nature of probability. Paulos observed[4] that many notions are as primitive as that of the barber who revealed his lottery strategy: 'The way I figure it, I can either win or lose, so I've got a 50–50 shot at it.'

24

Bradford Hill's doubts
(1993)

[T]he clinical trial must be as old as medicine itself. Even the witch-doctor trying out for the first time a new and nauseating compound must surely, like Alice nibbling at the mushroom in Wonderland, have murmured to himself, 'Which way?'

Bradford Hill[1]

Near the end of his life, Sir Austin Bradford Hill identified the most daunting challenge of his highly-esteemed career in biostatistics: to convince doctors 'there is not an unbridgeable gap between the statistical and clinical approach' to tests of any therapeutic procedure. Bradford Hill was unusually well suited to take on the challenge. He was very sympathetic to doctors' points of view because of his long interest in clinical medicine. (After a protracted bout of tuberculosis in World War I, he gave up all hope of a career in medicine; instead, he read economics and took the London University degree in 1922. He joined the statistical division of the National Institute for Medical Research in 1923.) Additionally, and equally significant, Bradford Hill had a life-long preference for plain language, and an aversion to technical jargon and verbosity. His determination to write clearly and succinctly stands out in an early series of papers that appeared weekly in the *Lancet* for the first four months of 1937.[2] When these articles (on the numerical approach to medical evidence) were published later that year in book form (*Principles of Medical Statistics*), the editor remarked on the author's 'exceptionally clear exposition of a difficult subject.' The handbook was quickly recognised as a classic; and, in edition after edition, it has been read for more than 50 years by successive generations of grateful medical students and doctors throughout the world.

For ten years after the appearance of his book, Bradford Hill looked for an opportunity to make a concrete demonstration of the need for a shift to experimental methodology (away from medicine's observations-only tradition) in tests of therapy. He had been arguing that the essential requirement in studies of the effects of interventions is concurrent comparison. This special need, he emphasised, stems from the important distinction between invariant events (relatively unusual in medicine), and variable phenomena that doctors deal with every day of their lives. '[I]n many respects the reactions of human beings are, under any circumstances extremely variable,' he wrote, '. . . and that is where the trouble begins.'

The opportunity for an instructive demonstration of the kind that he was looking for turned up just after the Second World War. In 1946, a small amount of the newly-discovered drug, streptomycin, was made available in Britain for the treatment of tuberculosis. A Committee of the Medical Research Council, spurred on by Bradford Hill, decided that a part of the small supply of the new drug should be used in a rigorously planned clinical investigation with concurrent controls.[3] The rest of the supply was used for treatment of two rapidly and uniformly fatal forms of the infection: miliary and meningeal tuberculosis. Since the outcomes in the latter disorders were invariable, Bradford Hill emphasised, there was no need for concurrent comparison with conventional management. If even one patient with proven meningeal or miliary tuberculosis made an indisputable recovery after treatment with streptomycin, 'should we not have a result,' he said, 'of the most profound importance.'

Pulmonary tuberculosis, on the other hand, was a perfect example of the very circumstance 'where trouble begins.' 'The natural course of pulmonary tuberculosis is. . . so variable and unpredictable,' the MRC Committee wrote, 'that evidence of improvement or cure following the use of a new drug in a few cases cannot be accepted as proof of the effect of that drug.' Bradford Hill recalled that Doctor Philip D'Arcy Hart, a distinguished expert in the field of tuberculosis, had been 'playing around with gold [in the treatment of pulmonary tuberculosis for 15 years] without being able to make a controlled trial and find out whether it was effective or not.'[4]

Fortunately, as it happened, Bradford Hill, D'Arcy Hart, and Marc Daniels (Hart's young assistant) were primed for the unusual opportunity provided by the arrival of streptomycin. They made a strong case for proceeding with an unprecedented multicentre randomised clinical trial without delay. 'It would *not* be immoral to make a trial,' they argued, 'it would be immoral not to make a trial, since the opportunity would never rise again (streptomycin would be synthesised, there would soon be plenty of it, so on and so on).'

The pioneering study, comparing streptomycin with conventional treatment (bed-rest), got under way in January, 1947. For enrolment and random allocation in this (if not the first, certainly most influential) experience, a prearranged order was determined by a table of random sampling numbers supplied by Bradford Hill; assignments were placed in sealed envelopes—separate sets were made up for male and female patients in each centre) continued until September, 1947. 'We could only have enough of the new drug to use on about 50 patients in the streptomycin arm of the trial,' Bradford Hill recalled, 'I thought that was probably enough to get a decent answer so long as [the trial] was strictly controlled and if streptomycin was really effective. And so it proved.'

Post-enrolment mortality indicated a clear advantage of the new treatment (4 deaths before the end of six months among 55 patients who received streptomycin versus 14 fatalities among 52 patients who were treated with bed-rest). The need for a control group in this study was underlined by the finding that impressive clinical improvement was seen in 13 patients treated by bed-rest alone. Important limitations of streptomycin treatment were also disclosed: the emergence of strepto- mycin-resistant strains of tubercle bacilli in a number of patients blunted the response to treatment, serious toxic effects of the new drug on vestibular function were encountered, and the drug appeared to have little effect on the chronic fibro-caseous forms of tuberculosis.

The streptomycin trial provided ample validation of Bradford Hill's arguments about the strength of experimental study-design. There was a striking contrast between the clear and quickly-obtained results of concurrent comparison, and the muddled status of gold treatment after 15 years of study without controls. The successful demonstration was a landmark in medical history. It led directly to the modern development of rigorous standards for the evaluation of therapeutic interventions.

The opportunity to make the convincing demonstration came about as the result of unique circumstances—the planners made a virtue out of scarcity. In later years, Bradford Hill wondered if permission to conduct the streptomycin trial would have been granted if there had not been a shortage of the new drug. 'I rather doubt it,' he mused, 'but I shall never know.' He was also doubtful that the streptomycin trial could have been carried out if the requirement for ethical committee oversight of informed consent (codified in the 1960s) had been in force in 1946. And, as noted earlier, he was dismayed to see an increasing trend to 'shift the entire consent-giving responsibility on the shoulders of patients who cannot really be informed or know what weight *relatively* to put on the technical information provided concerning risks and benefits.'

These frank words, written when Bradford Hill was in his 93rd year (about one and a half years before his death on 18 April 1991), called attention to the embarrassing gap between what is intended and what is, in fact, accomplished by the modern ritual of informed consent. A rigid policy has been in effect for more than 30 years, but there is very little firm evidence about the practical consequences of the 'shift of responsibility' that he recognised so clearly. It will be a fitting tribute to the memory of the inventor of the modern randomised clinical trial, if his criticism stimulates a much needed increase in the number of formal comparative studies of new approaches to informed consent in clinical trials.

(1997)

The uncomfortable gap between noble intention, and the crass everyday practice of obtaining informed consent has not been narrowed since Hill's comments. One impediment rests on the failure to establish an agreed-upon definition of the required elements of a consent doctrine— a reference standard to evaluate performance. This stumbling-block was identified a number of years ago by a lawyer and a psychiatrist; Meisel and Roth[1] proposed the following model for evaluating consent practices (the basic elements requiring specific definitions are italicised): '[W]hen *information* is disclosed by a physician to a *competent* person, that person will *understand* the information and *voluntarily* make a *decision* to accept or refuse the recommended procedure.'

Very few rigorous studies of the consent process had been undertaken, Meisel and Roth found, and, they concluded, 'There is very little wheat and much chaff.' Given the variety and extent of the deficiencies in published studies, they advised, 'it would be unwise to make law and policy on the basis of the available "facts".'

Unfortunately, little has changed. Recent observers charge[2] that 'there is a good deal of hypocrisy in clinical medicine about informed consent.' Many established treatments are poorly tested, their true benefits and risks are unclear, and, yet, these interventions are widely dispensed without the ritual of informed consent. 'Many more patients are exposed to this abuse of consent than in randomised controlled trials, but [the violations in everyday practice are] rarely questioned,' the writers observe. Preoccupation with the issue of informed consent in controlled studies 'will lead to fewer and smaller randomised trials and continued uncertainty over the risks and benefits of many treatments,' they conclude, ' and hence to continued widescale abuse of patients' consent in clinical practice.'

Bradford Hill pointed to the anomaly many years ago. He asked, 'Does the doctor invariably seek the patient's consent before using a new drug alleged to be efficacious and safe? If the answer is NO, then what process, one may ask, makes it needful for him to do so if he chooses to test the drug in such a way that he can compare its effects with those of the previous orthodox treatment?' Hill's question, Armitage recently observed,[3] has not 'yet received a convincing answer.'

25

More informative abstracts
(1993)

This paper isn't even good enough to be wrong.

Wolfgang Pauli[1]

More than a decade ago, Durack made a whimsical attempt to estimate the recent growth of medical knowledge by weighing the annual volumes of *Index Medicus* from 1957–1977.[2] (p. 26) Surprisingly, his rough curve paralleled the general form of increase for science as a whole predicted by Price:[3] a steady state of exponential growth followed by a decline to linear growth and, finally, an exponential rate of deceleration that approaches a 'saturation limit.' The slowing, if it has, in fact, occurred, is imperceptible to doctors confronted by the flood of new information that flows non-stop before their eyes in medical periodicals. Warren has noted[4] that a clinician must read about 200 articles and 70 editorials each month just to stay abreast of the current literature in internal medicine. It has been estimated[5] that a doctor, now caught-up and reading one article a day thereafter, would be, at the end of one year, 55 centuries behind in his/her reading!

Clinical epidemiologists at McMaster University in Canada have provided[6] a very sensible set of guidelines to help beleagured doctors separate the 'wheat from the chaff' in published articles with direct clinical applications. The selective approach is a pragmatic solution to the hopeless problem of trying to read everything, regardless of quality, published on a given topic.*

---

* The undiscriminating 'read everything' approach to medical literature is labelled 'looking for the pony.' The phrase, used by the Canadians, refers to a story they tell about two young boys, one of whom was an incurable pessimist, and the other an inveterate optimist. On Christmas Day, the young pessimist was given a room full of shiny new toys, and the optimist, a room full of horse manure. The pessimist opened the door to his room, sighed, and immediately complained about all of the shortcomings of, and problems brought on, by his new acquisitions. The optimist opened the door to his room and, with a whoop of joy, threw himself into the muck and began to dig in it. 'With all of this horse manure,' he exclaimed, 'there's *got* to be a pony in here somewhere!'

Early in the screening process, readers are advised to scan the 'Summary' or 'Abstract' section in a paper to decide whether the conclusion, if valid, would be of some practical use to them in everyday work. But, this precursory move to narrow the field is frustrated when there is no systematic format for summarising the contents of the article. The relevant information needed to make a quick decision about validity and applicability is, all too often, missing.

The need for uniformity in structure and in basic detail for abstracts of journal articles was recognised in 1969 by Ertl.[7] 'There is an urgent necessity to create a short form for presenting the contents of a publication,' he wrote, 'which would give a survey of the most important data, without the article having to be studied in detail.' His sensible proposal for a tabular presentation of seven important elements in articles (from '1. Formulation of question....' through '8. Complete results....') was not taken up by any medical journal. And there the matter rested for about 16 years until Brian Haynes, of McMaster University, approached the editor of *Annals of Internal Medicine*[8] to discuss the need for developing some mechanism that might improve medical readers' critical judgement concerning validity and applicability of conclusions reported in journal articles.

After lengthy discussions, that included recall of Ertl's neglected suggestion for structured abstracts, Haynes drafted a proposal for a new approach and sent it for comment to many interested persons throughout the world. The result of the efforts of this multi-national *ad hoc* group was published in 1987 as 'A proposal for more-informative abstracts of clinical articles.'[9] The group noted that the difficulties in using journals to help solve clinical problems are, to a considerable extent, logistical. Although modern electronic searching programs makes it possible to find applicable articles very quickly, the exploration 'is hampered by limitations of indexing and lack of systematic structure in the abstracts... of published articles, so that inclusion of seemingly appropriate terms in search statements both fails to retrieve all relevant articles and retrieves many that are not pertinent.' The solution to the information problem, the *ad hoc* group advised, 'is for authors of articles with direct clinical implications to prepare their abstracts so that key aspects of purpose, methods, and results are consistently described in a standardised manner with a *partially controlled vocabulary*' (italics added).

The key information proposed by the *ad hoc* group for selecting clinical articles of high relevance and quality was set out under seven headings:

'1. Objective: the exact question(s) addressed by the [study].

2. Design: the basic design of the study.

3. Patients or Participants: the manner of selection and numbers of patients or participants who entered and completed the study.

4. Interventions: the exact treatment or intervention, if any.
5. Measurement and Results: the methods of assessing patients and key results.
6. Conclusions: key conclusions including direct clinical applications.'

An important feature of the proposal—to improve the yield of computerised retrieval of relevant articles—appeared in an appendix in the form of a glossary of terms recommended for use by authors in preparing a structured abstract. Another proposal, for structured abstracts of review articles, was made in 1988 by Mulrow *et al.*[10]

Since publication of the 1987 and 1988 plans, a number of clinical journals have adopted the new format. Haynes and his co-workers report[11] that the US National Library of Medicine now includes structured abstracts in the MEDLINE file without modification or truncation despite their increased length (old style abstracts on MEDLINE are truncated at 250 words for articles less than 10 pages in length, and at 400 words for longer articles).

The outcomes of interest following implementation of the more-informative-abstracts format were stated by the *ad hoc* group in 1987: improvement in readers' ability to select articles that are valid and valuable, improvement of computerised literature searches, and facilitation of the peer review process. These objectives are testable and Haynes' group has drafted a research design to determine the extent to which the structured abstracts fulfil their hoped-for effects.

The approach may turn out to be useful in dealing with the acknowledged problems of choosing a limited number of papers for presentation at scientific meetings on the basis of the information provided in abstracts submitted by applicants. It is interesting to see that a few societies now require submission of structured abstracts for proposed papers and others may follow. But there need to be some systematic exploration of use of the scheme; and evaluation of the consequences of the change. For example, Does the structured abstract make it easier to make decisions about the quality of study design? Are the criteria for acceptance shifted from outcomes-based decisions to judgements based on methodological rigor of papers submitted for presentation?

(1997)

Following encouraging indications[1] that a structured format has had a positive impact on how information in abstracts is communicated, it became obvious there was a need to develop a similarly organised approach for the full texts in reports of randomised trials. A number of reviewers have complained that too many accounts of these exercises failed to provide readers with enough details about how the studies were carried out—the critical facts needed to judge the validity of many trials were conspicuous by their absence.[2] For example, the information given in 196 reports of randomised trials in rheumatology was so inadequate, Gøtzsche found,[3] 'it may be impossible to place any confidence in the statistical analyses or conclusions.' Similarly, there were indications that inadequate precautions against potentially biasing influences (unrevealed defects in design) were providing inaccurate estimates of the effects of interventions. As an example, Schulz and coworkers[4] reviewed 250 reports of randomised clinical trials (RCTs) and found suggestive evidence that trials in which the allocation sequence had been inadequately concealed were associated with relatively high estimates of treatment effects.

In 1994, two independent proposals were made for structured reporting of randomised trials.[2,5] Both argued that authors must provide sufficient valid and meaningful information concerning the design, conduct, and analysis of RCTs. Subsequently, a meeting was convened to reconcile the two proposals, and these deliberations led to a unified CONSORT statement (Consolidated Standards of Reporting Trials) published in 1996.[6,7] The agreed-upon proposal consists of a check-list of 21 descriptors that pertain 'to the methods, results, and discussion of an RCT report and identify key pieces of information necessary to evaluate the internal and external validity of the report.' Additionally, the proposal calls for a flow diagram that accounts for all eligible patients, and records their 'progress through all stages of a trial, including participants, withdrawals, and timing of primary and secondary outcome measures.' It is envisioned that every manuscript reporting trial results submitted for publication will now be accompanied by the CONSORT check-list, on which authors will note that each requirement was reported, and they will specify the page number in the manuscript where reviewers will find details of how each of the requisites was fulfilled.

The hopes for improved reporting based on the new standard are coupled with equally optimistic expectations that CONSORT will bring about improved planning and execution of RCTs. It is encouraging to see that several journals have now acted to require implementation of these rigorous standards.

26

Pain control in neonates
(1994)

An *infant* is, quite naturally, one who is unable to speak
(Latin: *in* = not + *fans*, speaking, from *fari*, to speak).[1]

Most parents have little difficulty in recognising their newborn infant's
cry of pain.[2] But there has been a prolonged debate among doctors about
the reliability and importance of this signal. The debate has reflected
discordant medical attitudes about pain and suffering that surfaced in
the mid-1800s when the vapours of sulphuric or diethyl ether, nitrous
oxide, and chloroform were found to abolish the pain of surgery.

Martin Pernick has reviewed the introduction and spread of the use of
the first anaesthetic agents in America; he found, surprisingly, a selective
pattern of application.[3] 'Many, if not most mid-nineteenth-century practitioners anaesthetised some of their patients and not others.' 'The issue for
them,' Pernick noted, 'was not whether to use anaesthetics, but when and
on whom.' Medical textbooks of the time taught that doctors should 'consider a patient's sex, race, age, ethnicity, economic class, personal habits,
and temperament . . . before using anaesthetic agents.' For example,
Pernick cited the opinion of Henry Bigelow, who published the first
article on the use of anaesthesia in 1848: 'The new technique is unnecessary for infants, because they lack the anticipation and remembrance of
suffering.' In 1852, Doctor Abiel Pierson of Massachusetts observed that
infants could sleep 'insensibly' even while undergoing surgery. Pierson
and others who believed in infant insensibility were convinced that the
ability to experience pain was related to intelligence, memory and rationality. 'Like lower species,' the doctors held, 'babies lack the mental capacity
to suffer.' Pernick reported that in an operation performed in 1854,
Samuel Cabot Jr., a colleague of Bigelow, wrote, 'the child patient was
rolled firmly in a sheet, as a substitute for ether.'

Others believed that the 'constitutions' of small children were such that
'the nervous power is . . . easily affected by stimuli,' and that babies were
extremely sensitive to pain. Pernick noted that some surgeons, notably
Samuel D. Gross and Eliza L.S. Thomas of the Women's College of

Pennsylvania in the 1850s, favoured the use of anaesthesia for infant patients. 'The young,' Doctor Thomas wrote, 'are innocents, unconscious of the motive for the surgery,' and they should be 'saved from suffering.'

A modern debate about the need for anaesthesia in very young babies undergoing surgical procedures erupted in 1986 with the publication of a letter in the US from a mother charging mistreatment of her premature infant.[4] Thoracotomy and patent ductus ligation had been performed without anaesthesia, the mother asserted; only oxygen and paralysing agents were administered during the $1\frac{1}{2}$ hour surgical procedure. Pain relief had been withheld, the mother was told, because 'it had never been demonstrated that babies can feel pain.' In answer to her complaint, an official of the American Medical Association wrote, 'Giving a premature infant the best chance to live is the primary medical objective; freedom from temporary pain is important, but it must be a secondary medical consideration.' These public arguments had the laudable effect of re-vealing that the practice of giving little or no analgesic and anaesthetic drugs to young babies undergoing surgery was very common in the US. According to the conventional wisdom, the risks of pain-relieving medi-cations were 'greatly multiplied' in infants—especially so in very small neonates.

A similar dispute exploded in Britain in 1987, following publication of an article by Anand and co-workers.[5] The paper had been awarded a prize the previous year as the best presentation by a young paediatrician at the annual scientific meeting of the British Paediatric Association. The prize-winning study, carried out in Oxford, was a small randomised trial (n = 16) of conventional anaesthesia (nitrous oxide and curare) com-pared with a new regimen (conventional anaesthesia plus intravenous fentanyl—a narcotic analgesic drug) for preterm infants undergoing liga-tion of a patent ductus. The researchers reported an important blunting of detrimental hormonal and catabolic responses to surgery in 8 infants who were operated on under the new anaesthetic regimen. And, Anand's group postulated, 'prevention of the massive stress response of preterm infants may lead to an improvement in their clinical outcome following surgery.'

The BPA[6] and other admirers of this ethically-sound, rigorously-designed, and very important challenge of a previously untested conven-tional practice, were astonished by loud charges of 'inhumane treatment' that followed publication of the article. The disapproval was voiced in letters to the editor ('How [could] an ethics committee approve [such] a study....?'[7]), in newspapers ('Pain-killer shock in babies operations'[8]), and in a press release signed by 14 MPs ('Inhumane baby operations slammed'[9]). Although the furor was distressing to the investigators, the complaints served a very useful purpose by calling public attention to the fact that long-accepted anaesthetic practices for small neonates must be questioned in considerable detail. (In a survey of British paediatric anaesthesiologists, 80% stated that they believed neonates were capable of feeling pain, and yet 48% never used narcotic analgesics and a further 41% seldom did so.[10]) The 1987 uproar also provided an unequalled opportunity to instruct members of Parliament about the propriety and validity of the modern randomised clinical trial format. Sir John Walton, president of the General Medical Council, replied to the Parliamentary group's charge that the study in question had been 'barbarous:'[11] 'I am persuaded after careful examination of the evidence before me that your concern is based upon certain serious misconceptions and a consequential failure to understand the true purpose and nature of this project and the treatment by anaesthesia, which it involved.' After a detailed rebuttal of each of the claims of impropriety, Sir John concluded, in unequivocal support of parallel-comparison studies of untested interventions, 'In my view, it would have been much more unethical for fentanyl to have been introduced without being submitted to the test of [a] randomised clinical trial.' On 17 September 1988, a public apology to the researchers was issued by a member of Parliament speaking for the Pro-Life critics.[12] 'It is now clear to me,' the spokesman stated, 'that the [trial] I criticised, far from being barbarous and unnecessary, [has] in fact been a valuable contribution to more humane treatment of preterm infants.'

The confidence in the serious intentions of the researchers and in the practical importance of the studies, expressed by supporters and, in the end, critics of the anaesthesia trial, has now been amply rewarded. Anand, now working with American co-workers in Boston, has reported the results of further studies of the dangerous responses of neonates triggered by major surgical operations. He and his associates have demonstrated that the hormonal and catabolic stress reactions of babies under-going surgical procedures is substantially greater than those of adult surgical patients.[13] And they have now completed a new randomised trial comparing the stress responses under two anaesthetic–analgesic protocols, of 45 critically ill neonates undergoing surgical repair of cardiac defects that required the use of cardiopulmonary by-pass and hypothermic circulatory arrest.[14] The two contrasting regimens of pain control were relatively light anaesthesia–analgesia (the conventionally-treated group received the usual doses of halothane and morphine) versus deep anaesthesia–analgesia (the experimental group received high doses of sufentanil [a potent opioid drug] and morphine). The very large hormonal-metabolic stress responses to cardiac surgery measured in the patients assigned to the light anaesthesia-analgesia regimen, were substantially reduced in the babies allotted to receive deep opiate anaesthesia–analgesia. Although pre-trial calculation of sample-size-needed was based on predicted difference in hormone and metabolic variables, the observed difference in clinical outcome (increased number of post-operative complications and number of deaths among infants assigned to the light anaesthesia-analgesia group) suggests that relatively deep levels of anaesthesia and analgesia may be required to improve post-operative outcome in critically ill neonates.

These disturbing findings confirm the darkest fears of many parents and nurses. The results cry out for additional observational and experimental studies by others to determine the extent to which the Oxford and Boston results can be generalised —particularly as they relate to the control of pain in all of the life-prolonging procedures carried out in neonatal intensive care. Anand and his co-workers, and now Quinn et al,[15] have let the genie out of the bottle: the issue of unrelieved pain and suffering in neonates can no longer be 're-bottled' and labelled 'a secondary medical consideration.'

(1997)

Quinn and co-workers (above) found that premature infants requiring ventilation and allotted to receive morphine by continuous drip, experienced reduced concentrations of adrenaline during the first 24 hours of treatment (as compared with an increase of adrenaline and noradrenaline among placebo-treated randomised controls). The observation that catecholamine concentrations were initially high and then fell in infants receiving opiate treatment, suggested to the authors that excessive stress, and perhaps pain, experienced by these infants, had been ameliorated by treatment. But no other differences in important outcomes were observed between the two groups in this trial; moreover, clinical signs of pain were similar in treated infants and in concurrent controls. Although the authors acknowledged that their findings did not make a strong case for routine use of morphine infusions in neonates undergoing ventilation, they concluded, as no significant adverse effects were found, 'it is humane to use a morphine infusion in babies who have to undergo ventilation for longer than 24 h.'

Wolf pointed out[1] other studies in infants and in adults, which demonstrated that 'stress responses are not directly linked to pain, and [therefore] stress hormones cannot be used as an indicator of adequate analgesia.' 'Limiting the stress response seems sensible,' he acknowledged, 'but the benefit in terms of outcome is difficult to prove.' Although opioids appear to be 'remarkably safe in critically ill babies,' he continued, 'tolerance develops rapidly.' 'Treatment of babies with large effective doses [of opiates] at times of major stress may therefore be more appropriate,' Wolf advised, 'than continuous infusions as long-term sedatives....'.

More trials are needed to settle the opiate-for-ventilated-neonates debate, nonetheless, the dramatic increase in awareness of the need for pain control in all neonates, indeed in all children, is both remarkable and heart-warming. A recent example of this modern avowal is seen in a survey of the use of opioid analgesia in one neonatal intensive care unit, when life support in critically-ill neonates was withdrawn or with-held.[2] Despite the potential of respiratory depression, the authors reported, neonatologists used these agents to relieve suffering in most of the dying infants (101 of 120 = 84%). Another example of the new sensitivity is found in a randomised trial testing the efficacy and safety of an analgesic cream used to control the pain of circumcision.[3] Similarly, 'pain services' have been established in some paediatric departments. One such multidisciplinary group was formed[4] to review the impediments to adequate pain management in childhood (dubbed 'The Ouchless Place'). The committee developed protocols for management of postoperative pain, uniform pain assessment, and for the blunting of pain in all needle procedures. The continued oversight, the authors pledge, will 'dramatically decrease the burden that illness imposes on hospitalised children and their families....'

The importance of these humane and long overdue advances cannot be overemphasised.

27

Miraculous cures
(1994)

I said that the cure itself is a certain leaf, but in addition to the drug, there is a certain charm, which if someone chants when he makes use of it, the medicine altogether restores him to health; but without the charm there is no profit from the leaf.

Socrates[1]

Many AIDS patients in the US have been enrolling, albeit reluctantly,[2] in a sizable number of controlled clinical trials testing more than seventy drugs meant to restore immune function or to treat AIDS-related infections. But clinicians conducting the trials have had a difficult time trying to explain to eligible patients why it is necessary to mask the identity of the drugs under test, and why caution is needed in deciding about cause and effect in these exercises. The importance of these issues was made clear in a revealing instance reported by Navarro.[3] An AIDS patient, enrolled in a formal trial, was overjoyed when he saw his CD4 cell count increase from 300 to 649. As a result, he urged his friends to buy the experimental drug as soon as possible on the black market. Encouraged by the sign of improvement, the patient began to take better care of himself, he ate three meals a day, and he began to exercise regularly. Then he found out he had been in the placebo arm of the trial: 'I was totally shocked,' he told the reporter, 'I thought it was the miracle drug.'

The AIDS incident is a reminder that the importance of expectation in determining response to treatment has been known for a very long time. For example, some of the most dramatic examples of the phenomenon were enacted on a very wide scale in Europe during the 18th century. The remarkable period began in 1766, Shorter recently recalled,[4] with Franz Anton Mesmer's thesis on graduating from medical school at the University of Vienna. In his dissertation, entitled 'The Action of Planets on the Human Body,' the budding doctor was influenced by Newton's theory of oceanic tides. He wrote about 'certain tides in the human body that might be accounted for by the movements of the sun and the moon' (then considered to be planets).

After graduation, Mesmer married a wealthy widow; he set up a medical practice in Vienna, and soon established a reputation for accepting difficult patients who had innumerable, hard-to-explain symptoms. Hilgard has noted[5] that the young doctor observed one such patient, Fräulein Oesterline, over an extended period, to see if the periodicity of her symptoms might fit in with his 'tidal' theory. On the assumption that the force of attraction exhibited by steel magnets was similar, somehow, to planetary action, Mesmer asked his patient to swallow a preparation containing iron. He then attached magnets to different parts to her body in an attempt to create 'artificial tides.' The patient described feeling 'streams of a mysterious fluid running within her body,' and she appeared to be cured of symptoms for several hours. Mesmer did not believe magnets alone had achieved the cure; he postulated that they merely reinforced the accumulation of a 'magnetic fluid' in his own body, and he named the phenomenon 'animal magnetism.' Repeated stroking motions with his fingers, Mesmer decided, transferred his ample supply of the invisible magnetic fluid to his patient, and she was eventually restored to health. The cure was reported in 1774, and other successes followed. The claims soon attracted a great deal of interest throughout Europe.

Mesmer moved to Paris in 1778, where his practice flourished. Sickness, he now believed, resulted from obstructed flow of the patient's magnetic fluid throughout the body. A therapist, with unusually strong 'magnetism,' could influence the distribution of the fluid by 'mesmerising' or massaging the body's 'poles.' The interaction often induced a crisis in the form of convulsions, and this was followed by the restoration of health. Darnton found a contemporary description of the dramatic performances put on by Mesmer and his followers:[6]

> [Mesmer's] method of curing a multitude of ills (among others, dropsy, paralysis, gout, scurvy, blindness, accidental deafness) consists in the application of a fluid or agent that M. Mesmer directs, at times with the end of his fingers, at times with an iron rod that another applies at will, on those who have recourse to him. He also uses a tub [filled with iron filings], to which are attached ropes that the sick tie around themselves, and iron rods, which they place near the pit of the stomach, the liver, or the spleen, and in general near the part of their bodies that is diseased. . . . There is a tub for the poor every other day. In the ante-chamber, musicians play tunes to make the sick cheerful. Arriving at the home of this famous doctor, one sees a crowd of men and women of every age and state. . . . It is a spectacle worthy of sensitive souls to see. . .

'Mesmerism has become an epidemic that has overcome all of France,' one observer wrote; 'The frenzy of mesmerism has overcome even the passion for balloon flights,' wrote another. The topic dominated the space in French journals for 1783–1784, the time of its greatest vogue. The movement was so serious that Louis XVI appointed a Royal Commission, in 1784, to investigate the claims of Mesmer and his followers. 'Never before in history,' Stephen Jay Gould has recently declared,[7] 'has such an extraordinary and luminous group of men been gathered in the service of rational inquiry by the methods of experimental science.' The commission consisted of four prominent physicians from the Faculty of Medicine (including Doctor Guillotin, who advocated use of the 'humane' execution machine that later came to be known by his name), and five members of the Academy of Sciences (including Antoine Lavoisier and Benjamin Franklin).

The commissioners observed the convulsions and trances of patients mesmerised by Charles Deslon, one of Mesmer's first converts; the investigators attempted to mesmerise themselves, without effect. They then tested the effects of Deslon's magnetic fluids, away from the excitable atmosphere of his clinic. For example, each of four cups of ordinary water were held before one of Deslon's patients in Lavoisier's home. The fourth cup produced convulsions; but the fifth cup of mesmerised fluid (believed by the patient to be plain water) produced no reaction. At another critical test in Franklin's garden, Deslon was asked to magnetise one of five trees. When a young man certified to be sensitive to magnetism, was asked to put his arms around each tree in turn, he fainted at the wrong tree.

After a number of additional tests—all failed to provide evidence for action of a magnetic fluid—the commission concluded that all claims of beneficial effects may be attributed to the power of imagination. 'The practice of magnetism,' they decided, 'is the art of increasing the imagination by degrees.' Gould quotes Lavoisier's important insight, recorded in the commission's report, about the lesson taught by the experience with mesmerism,

> The art of concluding from experience and observation consists in evaluating probabilities, in estimating if they are high or numerous enough to constitute proof. . . . The success of charlatans, sorcerers, and alchemists —all those who abuse public credulity—is found on errors in this type of calculation.

The frequent vogues of irrationalism in human history, Lavoisier concluded, are based on two hopes 'that touch [people] the most: that of knowing the future, and that of prolonging their days.'

The influence of expectation on a predicted event was of considerable theoretical interest to Karl Popper, the eminent epistemologist.[8] He named the confirming phenomenon, the 'Oedipus Effect' (after the causal chain leading to Oedipus' parricide that began with the oracle's prediction). But Popper encouraged a search for instances falsifying a prediction, as a solution to the problem of separating scientific statements from religious, metaphysical or pseudo-scientific declarations. His criterion of falsifiability holds that, 'statements or a system of statements, in order to be ranked as scientific, must be capable of conflicting with possible, or conceivable, observations.'

Popper would argue that the AIDS patient (above) should have been convinced about the scientific validity (and fairness) of the study design, when his expectation, that improvement was caused by 'the miracle drug,' was refuted. And the French Royal Commission was quite right to be more impressed by relatively few observations refuting the predictions of the animal magnetism movement, than they were by the thousands of testimonials in its favour.

(1997)

Jonathan Miller has recently written a very perceptive account1 of the intriguing historical link between Mesmer's animal magnetism and a later method to induce trance-like states—labelled 'hypnosis.' The damaging report of the French commission in 1785, Miller noted, was followed by a rapid decline of the mesmerism fad in that country. It flourished in England between 1786 and 1794; and then vanished from the scene, for a time, because of suspicion about anything associated with France. Animal magnetism reappeared in England in 1836, setting off 'scandalous high jinks' over the next few years; and this led to polarisation of professional opinion. Conventional doctors were divided between the true believers and others who scoffed at the claims; the latter were convinced patients' excited imaginations were at work in bringing about the theatrical 'cures.'

The stalemate was broken by James Braid of Manchester, Miller reported. Braid attended two demonstrations of animal magnetism in the early 1840s, and proposed the first ever, intelligible explanation of the patient's contribution to the phenomenon. On the second visit, Miller related,

> Braid noticed that the entranced subject was invariably unable to open his eyes, which led him to the belief that the trance was induced by something which he described as neuromuscular exhaustion induced by the protracted stare encouraged by the operator. To confirm this hunch he invited a friend...to gaze unblinkingly at the top of a wine bottle, as [the tyro experimenter] said, 'so much above him to produce a considerable strain on the oculomotor muscles.' Braid described the results in the following words, 'In three minutes his eyes closed, his head drooped, his face was slightly convulsed. He gave a groan and instantly fell into a profound sleep, the respirations becoming slow, deep and stertorous.

At the same time his right hand and arm were agitated by slight convulsive movements.'

Braid repeated the experiment, with the same result, on two other subjects (his wife and his man servant). 'He was convinced he had successfully demystified the mesmeric process. By formulating the concept of "nervous sleep," or hypnotism,' Miller reported, 'Braid developed a death blow to the pseudoscientific theory and supplied a more convincing alternative theory.' But, as it turned out, Braid was soon hoist by his own petard.

The experimenter soon discovered how easy it was to induce a hypnotic trance, and, before long, he was reporting dramatic cures of congenital deafness, hemiplegia, spinal curvature, ankylosing spondylitis, and epilepsy. As one reads about Braid's claims of conspicuous improvement in case after case, Miller observed, 'it begins to look as if the imagination of the physician is just as relevant to the outcome.' All too often, it seems, the excited imaginations of healers and their suffering supplicants lead to consensual delusions.

28

Observer bias
(1994)

How odd it is that anyone should not see that all observation must be for or against some view if it is to be of any service!

Charles Darwin

Before the explosive development of modern diagnostic technology, doctors took a great deal of pride in their ability to 'size up' their patients with a quick glance. On the basis of an unaided look-see, they often made Sherlock-Holmes-like deductions about details of their patients' lives and the nature of presenting complaints. The clinical exercise was made famous by one of Arthur Conan Doyle's teachers in medical school, Joseph Bell, an eminent Edinburgh surgeon. In May 1892, thirty-seven years after publication of *A Study in Scarlet*, the first Sherlock Holmes' detective story, Doyle wrote, 'I used and amplified [Bell's] methods when I tried to build up a scientific detective who solved cases on their own merits.'[1]

Bell developed a wide reputation for his skill as a keen observer. The surgeon's response to questions about his much admired talent, has been quoted by Wallace,

> The trouble with most people is that they see, but do not observe. Any really good detective ought to be able to tell, before a stranger has fairly sat down, his occupation, habits, and past history through rapid observation and deduction. Glance at a man and you find his nationality written on his face, his means of livelihood on his hands, and the rest of his story in his gait, mannerisms, tattoo marks, watch chain ornaments, shoelaces and the lint adhering to his clothes.

Bell's views on what he called 'the science of observation' made a lasting impression on five generations of medical students at Edinburgh University. One of the instructor's former pupils recalled a demonstration of the importance of paying attention to details; It took place in a packed amphitheater at the Royal Infirmary of Edinburgh. Bell held up a glass tumbler filled with an amber-coloured fluid, and told the students it was a potent drug with a very bitter taste. To investigate their perceptive abilities, he asked that they take part in a test. And, indicating he would not ask the students to do anything he himself would not do, he said, 'I will taste it before passing it around.' Bell dipped a finger in the fluid, put his finger to his mouth, sucked his finger tip, and grimaced. When the medicine was passed from hand to hand, each student dipped his finger into the fluid, sucked the finger tip, and, dutifully, made a wry face. When the round was completed, Bell looked out at his young audience, began to laugh; and then pointed out that not one of the students watched him closely enough to notice that Bell placed his forefinger in the bitter medicine, but he put his middle finger to his mouth!

Bell's views about the 'endless significance of trifles' were echoed by Doyle in story after story,[2] and he gave the Bell-cum-Holmes' cardinal rule for analysis and deduction: 'It is a capital mistake to theorise before one has data.' Although much admired in medicine, this facts-first-theory-later approach has perpetuated a myth about the supposed existence of unbiased (theory-free) observation.

Karl Popper criticised[3] the conventional view in lectures about a fundamental problem that must be taken into account when making any observation. He would stop his talk and challenge his students at the London School of Economics by asking, 'now carefully observe, and write down what you observe.' The students, confused by the request, asked, 'But what do you want us to observe?' Popper used the puzzled response to his directive to drive home a basic premise: 'No one can make a pure observation. First there must be a definite question in mind,' he emphasised, 'a theory that may be decided by the sense perceptions which follow.'

Popper,[4] and later Kuhn,[5] made a strong case for the proposition that all of our knowledge is theory-impregnated: theories come into being because of prior expectations. 'Joe' Bell was successful in distracting the students in his demonstration by leading them to expect they were participating in a taste test. And, in the clinics, Bell noticed details about patients that escaped the medical students because he looked with a theory-prepared, rather than an open mind. Moreover, the experienced surgeon used a limited number of 'off-the-shelf' theories; they were not constructed on the spot. One labourer's rough horny hands indicated to Bell that the man was a bricklayer; the calluses on the hands of another man were those of a carpenter, not a mason. Without these discrete 'theories,' the inexperienced students overlooked the clues, and the physical signs were meaningless until they were pointed out and explained by Bell.

Pattern recognition is, of course, a very useful skill, but significant limitations arise in the presence of novelty. Richard Asher was very interested in this shortcoming and he examined the problem in his famous Lettsomian Lectures before the Medical Society of London in 1959.[6] He showed a slide (Figure), at the beginning of the series of talks: it announced three topics to be discussed. Asher then developed the point that most people see what they expect, instead of seeing what is there. To bolster his argument, Asher disclosed that three gross errors in printing had been 'planted' in the slide—only one person in the large audience of doctors (Dr. Wilfred Oakley) picked out the intentional mistakes. 'We see what we expect,' he emphasised, 'and we unconsciously dismiss the anomalous.'

The clinician is both blessed and cursed by the suppressive mechanism,' Asher noted, 'blessed when he detects expected and significant patterns, but cursed when significant irrelevancies are tidied away without being appreciated.' As an example of how what we have been taught to see is much more important than how well we are able to see, Asher cited Francis Galton's experiment with sailors and landlubbers. Despite the fact that a group of men who had never been to sea and had better visual acuity than the old salts in the test, the sailors clearly outperformed the controls in spotting a distant mooring buoy. The men who lived on shore saw, Galton concluded, but did not notice; they perceived without recognising.

The relevance of these concerns about observer bias in all forms of scientific research is well known. Ederer notes the caution of a chemist:[7] 'The experimenter himself can be easily deceived in interpreting results, by his personal interest in the outcome.... No human being is even approximately free from these subjective influences.' And he cites an example of observer bias among laboratory technicians: The standard deviation of *masked* duplicate measurements of cholesterol was found to be considerably greater than that of *known* duplicate measurements in a large survey.

The stringent efforts made to reduce observer bias in formal clinical studies are often resented. But there is ample evidence to support the need for precautions. A recent example surfaced in a bitter dispute about the interpretation of findings in a controlled trial of treatment for otitis

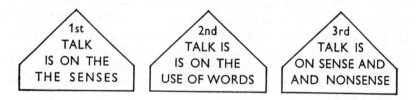

The lantern slide, announcing the topics to be discussed in Richard Asher's Lettsomian Lectures, contains three deliberate printing errors.

media with effusion.[8] The controversy turned on the issue of whether or not the expectations of observers accounted for a systematic difference between diagnoses of outcome made by tympanometry and by concurrent otoscopic examination. The conclusions of the trial concerning the efficacy of antibiotic treatment were challenged on the grounds that although the doctors examining the ears with an otoscope were said to be masked as to treatment received by each patient, 'some unknown factors such as reported side-effects or conversations with parents may have induced clues about assignment, thus influencing the observer (pp. 121–24).'[9]

It is insufficient to proclaim that a given study was 'masked,' Ederer warns, because the ideal is rarely, if ever, achieved. Investigators are always obliged to determine and to report the extent to which incomplete masking may have influenced the final results.

(1997)

The recent CONSORT statement (p. 105) calls for disclosure of specific details about 'masking.' In addition to descriptions about how the allocation sequence was generated in clinical trials (and then concealed until the patient has been randomised), authors are also required to provide 'evidence for successful blinding among participants, person doing [the] intervention, outcome assessors, and data analysts.'

The demand for these cloak-and-dagger-like dissimulations is often misunderstood—the requirement seems to imply that doctors cannot be trusted to act impartially. But it is completely unrealistic to expect that physicians have no prior expectations. Moreover, these understandable 'leanings' have practical consequences that may affect the results of a trial. The empirical evidence cited earlier (p. 105) supports the suspicion that prior knowledge of the next treatment (when the allocation sequence is poorly concealed) does influence a doctor's decision whether or not to enrol the next eligible patient. The need for concealment of the sequence of assignments cannot be overemphasised. It is also important to 'brand' patients indelibly (that is to say, outcomes should be tallied on the basis of 'intention to treat,' even when there are irregularities in the actual treatment received.

The need for elaborate precautions to hide all differences between a drug under-test and the concurrent control cannot be overstated. For example, in trials of psychotropic drugs, new agents are often compared with inactive placebos. The practice has recently been criticised by Greenberg and Fisher:[1] The easily detected side-effects of active drugs (e.g. dry mouth and constipation produced by antidepressant drugs) and the notable absence of such effects with a placebo, they point out, quickly unmasks the trial: patients and clinicians have no trouble spotting the enrolees who are, and others who are not, receiving 'real' treatment. And this transparency brings about inflated estimates of effect-size. In a small number of trials comparing antidepressants with an 'active placebo' (atropine, which produces a dry mouth) the difference in efficacy between the treated and controlled groups disappeared!

The warning voiced by Ederer more than 20 years ago, is reinforced by the experience in psychiatric studies: '...no drug trial should be considered acceptable,' Greenberg and Fisher caution, 'unless it contains measures of the degree to which the double mask has been broken.'

29

The gatekeeper's brouhaha
(1994)

> The evils of controversy are temporary, while its benefits are permanent.
>
> Reverend Robert Hall

A long-running *fin de siècle* melodrama in the US (mentioned briefly above) has, finally, played itself out. It has provided a revealing behind-the-scenes glimpse at the kind of machinations that can go on (rarely, one would hope) in the conduct and reporting of clinical trials. The cautionary tale, entitled 'The Cantekin Affair' by Drummond Rennie,[1] confirms the suspicion that temptations to circumvent the rules of evidence are particularly great when huge sums of money in drug sales depend on the outcomes of such trials. It also suggests that peer review of the quality of evidence generated in controlled clinical trials, even the surveillance maintained by the most prestigious medical journals, is weaker than we are willing to admit. When the affair was investigated by a US Congressional Subcommittee, the legislators were incensed; they asked, 'Are scientific misconduct and conflicts of interest hazardous to our health?'[2]

The episode (Robert Bell, in a very detailed examination,[3] refers to the sensation as the 'The Cantekin Dispute and the Bluestone Case') came to light when two manuscripts, reporting conflicting interpretations of the same set of data obtained in a 'double-blind, randomised trial', were submitted to the *New England Journal of Medicine* (one in June 1986, the other 4 weeks later). Both reported that a three-arm trial, conducted between July 1981 and October 1984 in Pittsburgh at the Children's Hospital Otitis Media Research Center, compared the effects of amoxicillin plus decongestant-antihistamine, amoxicillin plus placebo, and placebo alone in 518 children with 'secretory' otitis media (otitis media with effusion).

The editor of *NEJM* wrote to the University of Pittsburgh School of Medicine and to the Children's Hospital to ask which of the two manuscripts was the 'official' version. Both institutions replied that Dr. Charles Bluestone, a well-known otologist and principal investigator of the study under consideration, and Dr. Ellen Mandel, the lead author, were the only persons authorised to report the results. This 'official' version was then duly reviewed. Bell notes, that the editors asked the authors to 'tone down' the conclusion (which read, 'amoxicillin is effective and should be used in the treatment of secretory otitis media in children'). An amended version of the report was published in February 1987;[4] readers were told that 'amoxicillin increases to some extent the likelihood of resolution [of "secretory" otitis media].'

The 'maverick' manuscript (which concluded that 'amoxicillin ... is not effective ') was returned without review. The editor of *NEJM*, Bell reports,[3] gave a surprising reason for rejecting it: 'The important question ... is not whose interpretation is correct ... but who has the right to publish ...!' (Later in the dispute, a lawyer wrote to the editor and said, 'Let me reword your statement just slightly to demonstrate its astonishing absurdity: "The important question ... is not whether Galileo or the Pope is correct with respect to whether the sun revolves around the earth or vice versa, but rather, who, as between the Pope and Galileo, has the right to publish his opinion. ..."')

Disagreement between the two protagonists, Bluestone and Erdem Cantekin (a bioengineer, who was Director of Research in the Department of Otolaryngology) began even before completion of the RCT in question. The Research Center, established in 1980 with a US$12-million National Institutes of Health (NIH) grant, was also receiving money from pharmaceutical companies; this led Cantekin, in June 1983, to express doubts about 'the scientific validity of research commissioned by and funded by pharmaceutical companies seeking to prove the effectiveness of their antibiotics.' He argued that the Center should disassociate itself from industry-sponsored studies. Cantekin also charged that the principal investigator 'was publicly advocating the use of amoxicillin for "secretory" otitis media before the trial was over ... he [Bluestone] spent substantial time travelling at the expense of the pharmaceutical company to advocate use of their product.'

When the amoxicillin-trial was concluded in 1984, drafts of a manuscript were circulated. Bell reports that Cantekin disagreed with the conclusion about effectiveness of the drug; in September 1985, he bowed out as a co-author 'on the thirteenth draft of the paper.' He then asked two experts in the analysis of data to join him, and they wrote the 'maverick' version of the report that was rejected without review by *NEJM*. In August 1986, shortly after the unauthorised paper was submitted for publication, Cantekin was discharged from his position at the Center. According to a hearing board of the medical school, he had committed 'serious violations of research ethics.' For the next few years, Cantekin wrote letters to the dean of the medical school, to NIH, to the Food and Drug Administration, to the US Congress, and to the editors of medical journals to press his complaints of a conflict of interest and of misrepresentation of the results of the amoxicillin-trial. He tried, without success, to have the 'maverick' paper published. A series of investigations, including two hearings before a subcommittee of the US Congress,[2] took place in which all parties traded charges and counter-charges. What emerged from all of the debate was grudging acknowledge-ment that there was some substance to the criticisms levelled against the 'official' version of the amoxicillin-trial.

For example, this publication[4] failed to provide an explanation of how sample-size-needed was calculated before the trial began; and there was no mention that the trial was, in fact, terminated prematurely. Later investigation revealed that the trial was stopped arbitrarily after the enrolment of 518 children, before reaching the original target sample-size of 1040 subjects. Cantekin explained[5] that 'this early termination was not based on any sound statistical criterion;' the Center had a deficit and 'it was desperate to obtain an infusion of money from private pharmaceutical companies.' Funding from two companies was obtained and a new trial evaluating another antibiotic was started without inform-ing NIH (which continued to fund the program) of the change. Later investigation by NIH noted, 'We find merit to the allegation that [the Research Center] has not disclosed to NIH the extent of its industry-sponsored research.' Bluestone admitted to the congressional subcom-mittee that by 1989, the amount of the drug-company funding totalled US$3.5-million.

Cantekin pointed out that the amoxicillin-study protocol specified that the primary outcome was to be the proportion of children without effusion 4-weeks after beginning treatment. As specified before the trial began, the decision was to be based on a diagnostic algorithm which took into account otoscopic and tympanometric changes, and a test of hear-ing. However, in a congressional hearing, it was found that the algorithm used in the 'official' analysis of results was not the one described in the original study protocol; and NIH was not notified of the change of diag-nostic criteria for the primary outcome. Cantekin found a systematic difference between the 'objective' findings of secretory otitis (based on tympanometry and on hearing tests) and the 'subjective' signs (otoscopic changes as judged by the otologists). The efficacy of amoxicillin, Cantekin argued, was relatively inconsequential 'by all outcome measures that are not heavily influenced by otoscopy.' A panel of scientists,[6] convened by NIH's Office of Scientific Integrity, concurred; they found that the data at 4 weeks provided 'no real evidence' that antibiotic therapy was superior to placebo.

Another issue emerged in the investigations, Bell has noted: the 'cure' rate in the placebo arm of the amoxicillin-trial was half the rate found in other studies of secretory otitis media. The unusually low rate of spon-taneous improvement had the spurious effect of making an otherwise unexciting amoxicillin-treated-rate-of-cure look important. Cantekin charged that even though the Center was aware of higher placebo-rates-of-cure reported in other published studies (as well as a higher placebo-cure rate in the Center's own antibiotic trial undertaken immediately after the amoxicillin study), the anomalous finding was glossed over in the 'official' publication.

When the 'maverick' version of the trial was finally published in December 1991,[7] Rennie wrote an accompanying editorial[1] in which he reviewed the tortuous details of the controversy, and addressed the question, 'Why has it taken so long for this article to see the light of day?' In retrospect, he mused, it might have been wise to publish both manuscripts and leave it to the reader to decide between them. This solution (it might be dubbed 'the Cantekin resolution,' Rennie suggested) 'would have best served the cause of scientific openness.' And he added, 'It would surely have provoked a lively correspondence: in many ways the very best form of peer review.'

Secretory otitis media is an extremely costly medical problem in the US. In 1980, the disorder accounted for 5 million visits to the doctor by American children under 3 years of age; the annual cost is estimated to be US$1 to 2 billion.[8] When such high stakes are involved, Bell has concluded, the journal review process fails to detect error due to conflict of interest. Moreover, the gatekeepers (department chairs, institutional review boards, editors), who control the flow of information that passes before the eyes of doctors on the front lines, seem to abhor controversy more than they love the truth. If this dour judgement about the weak safeguards to ensure integrity in present-day drug trials is correct, it suggests, among other things, that the lessons of past drug disasters (thalidomide, diethylstilbestrol. . .) are fading from memory. Unfortunately, as Santayana observed, 'Those who cannot remember the past, are condemned to relive it.'

(1997)

The stakes involved in the introduction of new treatments have become enormous. For example, in 1990 an advisory panel of the US Food and Drug Administration declined to recommend approval of interleukin-2 as an anticancer agent. The decision, Hall has reported,[1] 'led directly to the demise of Cetus Corporation, the molecule's manufacturer.' The company's capitalisation was US$1-billion in 1986; it ceased to exist by the end of 1991. The company had gambled its entire survival on the regulatory agency's approval.

The FDA's powerful gatekeeping function, Dreyfuss recently explained,[2] has made it the target of well-financed battles to diminish the agency's role as 'a strong and independent guardian of America's health.' For instance, loud complaints about the slow pace of testing new drugs in the US led to passage of the Prescription Drug User Fee Act in 1992. The enabling legislation authorised the hiring of additional staff at the FDA to speed-up evaluations. Over a period of 5 years, more than US$300-million was made available to hire 600 new personnel, and the time needed to carry out the final phase of the approval process was cut nearly in half.

These generous funds, generated by levies on pharmaceutical companies, have come to provide a relatively large fraction of the FDA's total budget. So much so, Dreyfuss noted, that the agency has been negotiating directly, but quietly, with drug and biotechnology companies for 'reforms' in exchange for the industries' support to continue the subsidies in a reauthorised Professional Drug User Fee Act (the 1992 law was set to expire in 1997). Among the 'reforms to modernise' the gatekeeping function of the FDA, the drug companies seek changes in procedures that 'would speed up the clinical trials phase of the drug approval process by 10 to 16 months (an acceleration that could mean hundreds of millions of dollars to companies able to market their products much sooner'). Additionally, the industry wants legal sanction to allow companies to promote their products for uses that are not specifically approved by the FDA—so-called 'off-label use.' Medical device companies are lobbying for increased use of 'outside reviewers' (allowing the FDA to contract out its review of new devices to so-called 'independent scientific review organisations'), and the industry seeks legislation that would ensure a company's 'immunity from lawsuits if a faulty product had previously secured FDA approval.'

If these machinations continue, Dreyfuss warns, 'the FDA could find itself facing a runaway piece of legislation that would compromise fundamental parts of its mission.'

30

Creatures of bounded rationality
(1995)

It is always thus, impelled by a state of mind which is destined
not to last, that we make our irrevocable decisions.

Marcel Proust[1]

Prior to the therapeutic explosion in the modern era, there was relatively
little interest in the process by which doctors went about making decisions to use the largely ineffective remedies available throughout most
of medicine's long and colourful history. As interventions have become
more effective in altering the natural course of disease, the topic of
decision-making by doctors, and, increasingly, by their patients and
surrogates, needs to be explored in detail. Decisions which lead to
important consequences, social scientists now recognise, are usually
made reluctantly. 'We see [the human decision-maker] not as a cold fish,'
Janis and Mann have written,[2] 'but as a warm-blooded mammal; not as
a rational calculator always ready to work out the best solution, but as
a reluctant decision-maker—beset by conflict, doubts, and worry,
struggling with incongruous longings, antipathies, and loyalties, and
seeking relief by procrastinating, rationalising, or denying responsibility
for [his/her] own choices.'

As noted earlier (p. 95), there is growing interest in a 'restaurant model'
for shared decision-making in medicine. Doctors provide patients or
surrogates with updated estimates of the probabilities of outcomes-of-
interest for each of the treatments on the 'menu;' patients or surrogates
decide on which of the proposed courses of action will lead to the outcomes they prefer. But problems arise when those whose lives and well-
being are at-risk, make crucial choices that seem to be patently unsound
from their physicians' point of view. As it turns out, investigations of
the psychology of preferences[3] have demonstrated that discrepancies
between objective and subjective conceptions of the right-mindedness of
decisions occur frequently.

Interest in departures from the objectivity of preferences is thought to
have started in 1738 with the observations of Daniel Bernoulli, a Swiss

mathematician and physician, when he tried to explain the paradoxical behaviour of gamblers.[4] His observations led him to argue that 'the *emolumentum* [worth] of the ducat a gambler gains is smaller than the *emolumentum* of the ducat he loses.' Bernoulli's argument was overlooked until Jeremy Bentham formulated a similar principle in 1802 called the Principle of Decreasing Marginal Utility: 'For any given individual, each additional unit of money or commodity increases utility by a decreasing amount.'

Modern investigations have confirmed that in many situations a decision seems to be influenced more by the threat of a loss than by the possibility of an equivalent gain. There is heightened sensitivity, it seems, to the difference between certainty and high probability, but relative insensitivity to intermediate gradations of probability. Tversky and Kahneman ask us to imagine, for example, that we are given a choice between two options. The first is a sure gain of £80. The second option offers an eighty-five-percent chance of winning £100 and a fifteen-percent chance of winning nothing. Most people presented with this choice, they found, prefer the certain gain to the gamble, despite the fact that the gamble has a higher 'monetary expectation' than the assured outcome. (The monetary expectation reflects the average monetary value of the gamble: If the gambling option is exercised repeatedly, the average gain is calculated to be about £85 per play.) 'A choice is risk-*averse*,' they conclude, 'if an absolutely certain outcome is preferred to a gamble with an equal or greater monetary expectation.'

On the other hand, a consequential choice is considered 'risk-*seeking* if a certainty is rejected in favour of a gamble with an equal or lower monetary expectation. In the example given by Tversky and Kahneman, we are asked to choose between an unequivocal loss of 80, and a gamble that involves an 85 per cent chance of losing £100 and a 15 per cent chance of losing nothing. Faced with this choice, they observed, a substantial majority prefer the gamble rather than the certain loss, even though a calculation of the probabilities demonstrates that the monetary expectation of the gamble (−£85) is worse than that of the sure loss (−£80).

The pattern that emerges from these studies of hypothetical problems —and others involving choices such as duration of pain, the number of lives lost in an epidemic, or prolongation of life by medical intervention—seem to be consistent. Preferences between gains are most often risk-averse; preferences between losses are usually risk-seeking.

The insights provided by studies of the way people make risky choices in everyday life are of particular interest in trying to understand the kind of mismatched attitudes that may arise at the birth of a marginally-viable VLBW (very low birth weight) infant. The objective view of a team of neonatologists and the subjective outlook of parents may be completely incongruent. There is a strong suspicion that the discord is brought about by what are termed 'framing effects:' preferences for medical action are dependent on how the outcomes are perceived. The rescue team advises aggressive treatment on the basis of objective evidence from surveys that the prognosis for unimpaired survival is good (probability of disability is '25%, confidence interval 21–30%'[5]). Parents who refuse heroic measures focus on the long-term consequences of losing the gamble. Here the outcome is framed in terms of parents' subjective fears: the frightening prospect of an unrelieved physical and financial burden that will fall on the entire family who may need to provide care for a severely disabled child from early infancy to adult life; the intense guilt, rage, bitterness, shame, stigma, and frustration many parents experience in a demanding role to which they feel they have been unfairly assigned—a part they feel poorly equipped to play.

Nobelist Herbert Simon has demonstrated,[6] that, on the whole, decision-makers pursue a strategy which he calls satisficing, when they are required to make hard choices; that is to say, they look for a course of action that is 'good enough,' a decision that meets a minimal, rather than an exhaustive, set of requirements. The superficial approach fits the limited information-processing capacities of human beings. 'The world,' Simon argues, 'is peopled by creatures of "bounded or limited rationality," and these creatures constantly resort to gross simplifications when dealing with complex decision problems.'

As perinatal/neonatal medicine's technical achievements become increasingly more miraculous, doctors and parents are faced with choices which are increasingly obscure, complex and far-reaching in their implications. The process of decision-making under these never-before-encountered conditions cries out for systematic study.

(1997)

Framing effects, of the kind described above, also appear to play a part in choices made by doctors and other health-care professionals. 'Clinicians are much impressed by the bigger numbers of relative changes,' Feinstein has opined,[1] 'than by the smaller magnitudes of the absolute changes for the same results.' Fahey and co-workers set out to explore this thesis in Britain several years ago:[2] Are 'health policy decisions influenced,' they asked, 'by the way in which results of clinical trials and systematic reviews are presented?'

Postal questionnaires were sent to 182 executive and non-executive members of the various regional health authorities and commissions responsible for setting health policy, for purchasing and for other administrative matters related to health in the Anglia and Oxford regions; 140 of the forms were returned. The questionnaire was constructed to report the actual data from two studies (a clinical trial of the efficacy of breast cancer screening, and a systematic review of the efficacy of cardiac re-habilitation). The true results for each programme were presented in four different ways: (i) as a relative risk reduction; (ii) an absolute risk reduction; (iii) as the proportion of event-free patients; and (iv) as the number of patients-needed-to-treat to prevent one death. The researchers found that 'Health authority members' willingness to purchase services was influenced by the methods used to present results.' They appeared to be 'more impressed by measurements that report relative benefits compared with those entailing an index of absolute benefit.' (Interestingly, only three respondents [all non-executives, claiming no training in epidemiology] said 'they realised that all four sets of data summarised the same results.')

Among other implications of these findings, Milne and Sackett commented,[3] 'purchasers may also need a programme of skills development to ensure that when charged with basing decisions on evidence, they know how to make sense of that evidence.' Evidence-based medicine has its work cut out!

31

Champing at the bit
(1995)

'Begin at the beginning,' the King said gravely, 'and go on till you come to the end: then stop.'

Alice's Adventures in Wonderland

The decision to end patient enrolment in the pioneering streptomycin trial in 1947 (p. 100) was dictated by the very small supply of the new agent then available for treating pulmonary tuberculosis. 'We could only have enough of the new drug to use on about 50 patients in the streptomycin arm of the [randomised] trial,' Bradford Hill explained. Later, planners began to calculate the number of patients needed for RCTs based on several pre-trial stipulations (p. 12): an unambiguous definition of the primary outcome of interest, the smallest treatment difference in this outcome that would be considered too important to miss, and the degree of certitude in asserting at the conclusion of the trial that there was, or was not, an important difference between the compared treatments. These early fixed-sample-size trials were carried out with the understanding that the results were not to be inspected until the trial was completed. The restraint was necessary, it was argued, to reduce the error of declaring a 'winner' too soon—as in the fabled race between the hare and the tortoise, early trends can be very deceptive.

Before too long the 'no peeking' rule in fixed-sample-size clinical trials ran into an unacceptable difficulty. For example, in 1954 a trial was carried out in America[1] to determine whether a newly-recommended antibacterial drug (oxytetracycline) was more effective than the standard regimen (penicillin plus sulfisoxazole) for small neonates. Prophylactic treatment of these vulnerable infants was necessary, it was felt, because of a high risk of fatal infections that were difficult to diagnose. In planning the size of the comparative trial, it was decided that a reduction in first-five-day mortality to 25% (from 37% experienced the previous year) would be an important result that should not be missed. This meant that a fixed sample size of about 100 infants in each treatment group would be required to be reasonably confident (95% level) of a verdict in favour of the new agent.

The trial excited very little interest among the caretakers; the staff (including pathologists) had no difficulty in resisting any temptation to 'peek' at the results before the trial was completed. As the trial was drawing to a close, two young doctors studying the relationship between peak serum bilirubin concentration during life and kernicterus at postmortem, stumbled onto the fact that most of the examples of kernicterus were found in infants who received penicillin/sulfisoxazole prophylaxis. The trial results were then quickly examined (192 of a planned total of 200 infants had been enrolled): the findings were so shocking the study was stopped immediately. The difference in early-mortality rate between the two treatment groups was much higher than predicted when planning the dimensions of the trial. Although infants allotted to the *established* regimen (penicillin/sulfisoxazole) did have fewer fatal infections, this hoped-for beneficial effect was irrelevant: Infants receiving the standard prophylaxis died at more than twice the rate observed in the oxytetracyclene-treated infants. The increased mortality seemed to be accounted for by kernicterus—a completely unexpected association (the causal reasoning was made plausible later when sulfisoxazole was shown to induce lethal kernicterus in jaundiced newborn rats).

Although the researchers took some comfort in the knowledge that one-half of the infants enrolled in the trial had been protected from a previously unrecognised hazard of an accepted and widely used treatment, it was clear that a definitive difference in the comparative study could have been recognised, and the trial stopped, much earlier if on-going results had been monitored closely.

The experience in the sulfisoxazole trial, and other trials that revealed unexpected complications, led directly to the development of sequential designs for 'continuous peeking;' and to the use of independent monitoring committees to conduct interim analyses of results (with appropriate statistical corrections for multiple tests on accumulating data), and they were charged with the responsibility of looking for unexpected harmful effects in on-going clinical trials. In recent years, close oversight has created its own set of problems. There are increasing pressures on trialists, Miké has noted,[2] to stop enrolling patients when preliminary trends become apparent—before the study design calls for termination of the trial.

The demands for smaller trials and prompt release of interim data have come from some ethicists and from patients-rights activists. The critics seem unwilling to accept the implications of an immutable fact of life: Large numbers of replications are required in deciding about cause and effect in medicine because the responses of human beings to interventions are, on the whole, extremely variable. 'And that,' Bradford Hill once remarked about this fundamental issue, 'is where the trouble begins.' As noted previously, one ethicist has declared (p. 38) that physicians have a *therapeutic obligation* to stop enrolment as soon as 'a trial has reached a stage such that the hypothesis that therapy A is inferior to therapy B is more probable than its opposite. . . .' He conceded that '[A]doption of this rule would greatly increase the incidence of false positive results in clinical trials,' but, he concluded, there is an insurmountable 'ethical argument against continuing a trial until definitive results are achieved.'

AIDS activists have been particularly impatient with the slow process of drug evaluation in large-scale trials needed to provide reliable estimates of effect-size and magnitudes of risks in proposed therapies. The impatient demands for a 'fast track' approach in America led to the use of a surrogate marker (improvement in CD4 cell count) in symptom-free HIV-infected patients to measure a beneficial effect of treatment quickly. For example, four relatively-small controlled trials in the US indicating the effectiveness of the zidovudine (AZT) for such patients relied on improvement of the cell marker, and on relatively short-term estimates of progression to symptomatic disease as the outcomes of interest. Three of the four studies were terminated early with average follow-up of about one-year or less; in the fourth, follow-up was just over two years. Now the significance of these short-term results, used to obtain an American licence, has been challenged.

The clamour to speed up licensing of new agents seems to have come a cropper with the recent publication of a letter summarising results of the Concorde trial of AZT.[3] This large-scale multicentre controlled trial (comparing immediate treatment of symptom-free HIV-infected patients versus deferring treatment to the onset of symptomatic disease) was conducted in the UK, France and Ireland; the report was based on 5 328 person-years of follow-up (mean follow-up three years). The endpoints in the tri-country trial were progression to symptomatic disease, severe drug toxicity and death. There had been pressure to end the trial ahead of schedule when early analysis of a similar American study of AZT demonstrated drug-related improvement. Some critics charged that continuation of the Concorde trial was unethical, but the researchers pressed on. 'They did not believe the American study had continued long enough to resolve the issue of whether AZT might give short-term benefits, but fail in the long term.'[4] As it turned out the Concorde group found that benefits observed in the first few months (as judged by CD4 counts) were short-lived. In the long-term, no benefit could be demonstrated from the immediate use of AZT in symptom-free individuals, in terms of survival or disease progression. The researchers concluded that the discrepancy between this result and the cell-count-based optimism about the effectiveness of AZT casts doubt on value of using changes in the surrogate marker over time as a predictive measure of drug effectiveness.

The lesson of the AZT experience, Ian Weller, leader of the British team, has warned, is this: 'Don't stop trials too early.' Iain Chalmers, Director of The UK Cochrane Centre in Oxford, has also commented on the instructive turn of events: the Concorde findings are 'a needed challenge to those of us who conduct trials,' he noted. 'There is so much money to be made in approving new drugs, the pressure to approve is great. What needs to be determined,' he emphasised, 'is whether people conducting trials are actually measuring things that matter.'

(1997)

There has been no easement in the difficulties faced by Data Safety and Monitoring Committees when they must decide before pre-planned times of completion, to stop enrolment in high profile clinical trials of risky treatments. There are no easy solutions to the opposing-interests dilemma—the present stake of trial participants versus the welfare of future patients in similar straits. The predicament is sharply defined, Singer points out,[1] when the clinical usefulness of a proposed treatment depends on a 'fine quantitative balance between net efficacy and net toxicity.'

The complex issues were highlighted in the experience with controlled trials of long term anticoagulation in patients with atrial fibrillation who are at increased risk for cerebral stroke (this complication accounts for sizeable morbidity in the elderly). Five RCTs of anticoagulation with the drug 'warfarin' were carried out in the 1980s, Singer reports, and 'all five stopped early because of marked reduction in the rate of stroke in groups treated with warfarin.' But relatively few events were recorded in each trial and, as a consequence, confidence intervals for the estimates of the benefit were very wide. Thus, the decisions of millions of at-risk individuals throughout the world to begin life-long warfarin were dependent on very imprecise evidence.

For example, Singer writes that by the fifth year of study the Boston Area trial recorded a striking reduction of strokes in warfarin-treated patients, and these anticoagulant-treated patients experienced no apparent increase in major bleeding. But the total number of strokes in this trial was only 15 (13 in 435 person-years of observation among controls, and two strokes in 487 person-years in the warfarin arm). The point estimate of the protective effect was an impressive 86%, but this was blurred by the wide confidence interval ranging from 51% to 96% .

It can be argued that this imprecision in the estimate of benefit was of no practical importance, because no increase in major bleeding was observed in trial-patients treated with warfarin. However, as Singer explains, only a small proportion of the total number of at-risk patients were enrolled in the Boston trial and, he suspects, they were a select sample of that whole population: 'patients recruited into the trial were less likely to bleed and more likely to comply with frequent prothrombin time measurements than the average [at-risk] patient. . . . ; [before enrolment] patients were explicitly screened for bleeding risks, and more informally screened for the ability to comply with the trial's schedule of monitoring.' Following completion of the trials , he reports, 'real world' observations of warfarin's toxicity indicated relatively high rates of major bleeding.

Overly cautious stopping rules, when applied to risky therapies, Singer opines, 'short change the interests of the greater [target] population.' And the counter argument (very high thresholds for stopping rules place trial participants at unacceptable risk) is weakened, he concludes, when participants have a chronic disorder that persists after completion of the trial. Here, 'participants have a stake in maximizing the information generated by trial(s) since that information will benefit their own treatment when they return to standard clinical practice.'

32

Piecemeal skirmishes
(1995)

Each time we learn something new and surprising, the astonishment comes with the realisation that we were wrong before.... In truth, whenever we discover a new fact it involves the elimination of old ones. We are always, as it turns out, fundamentally in error.

Lewis Thomas

An American ophthalmologist, Theodore Terry, described the first known instance of retinopathy of prematurity (ROP) in 1942,[1] and he speculated that '...some new factor has arisen to produce such a condition.' Fifty-years later, John Watts carried out a rigorous review of the evidence that has accumulated in efforts to solve the five-decades-old mystery.[2] There has been a persistent hope that Terry's single 'new factor' will be uncovered and an expectation that ROP-blindness in prematurely-born infants will be completely eliminated. But this optimism, Watts makes it clear, is unwarranted. '[N]ot only are we still severely limited in our ability to prevent, treat or even understand the disease,' he writes, 'but the problem may be increasing.'

What stands out in the search for a solution to the puzzle presented by the unique retinopathy, is how disjointed the pursuit has been. There have been many leads, but very few have been tested rigorously in large-scale experimental trials. For example, only two large multicentre randomised trials were carried out in the fifty-year history of the disorder. The first of these exercises was conducted in the US in 1953–54,[3] to evaluate the effect of modifying the accepted liberal policy of administering oxygen in the care of prematurely-born infants ('routine' use of high concentrations of the life-sustaining gas to all infants weighing less than 1.5 kg at birth). The trial demonstrated that the relative risk of cicatricial retinal lesions could be reduced about two-thirds by using the gas 'only as needed;' but the curtailment of oxygen did not totally eliminate the risk of blindness.

The second multicentre randomised trial, carried out thirty-two years later,[4] tested the safety and efficacy of trans-scleral cryotherapy in halting the progression of moderately advanced acute ROP in infants weighing less than 1.25 kg at birth. The ablative procedure reduced the expected rate of unfavourable retinal outcome by one-half; but, again, the intervention did not completely eliminate the risk of blindness.

An early example of the kind of endless speculation about the sole necessary and sufficient cause of ROP is the on-going debate about the putative role of light; it began with Terry in 1942. A number of studies have been carried out to determine whether or not exposure to the high level of ambient fluorescent light commonly found in present-day nurseries increases the risk of ROP, but the studies have been much too small and the study-designs have been too weak to provide reliable estimates of the size of a purported light-effect. Despite five-decades of interest and repeated claims about the causal role of light, the matter remains completely unsettled. And the same must be said about all other plausible-but-never-fully-tested influences on the origin and the course of ROP.

The 45 year-old history of the testable-notion that vitamin E might prevent ROP is another unhappy example of the never-fully-tested problem that has resulted in such intractable uncertainty. In 1949, Owens and Owens suspected that a relative lack of vitamin E might play a causal role in the development of the retinopathy, and they began a small, open (not masked) trial of prophylactic treatment using concurrent untreated controls.[5] The early trend in favour of vitamin E was so impressive the senior advisors in the department of ophthalmology ordered the young husband and wife team to abandon the trial; and prophylactic vitamin E was then given to all premature infants admitted to the premature nursery. Several observational studies in other centres were unable to confirm the earlier results indicating a protective effect of vitamin E; soon all interest in this agent evaporated. In the 1980s, there was renewed interest in the efficacy of vitamin E (now it was the anti-oxidant property of this substance that captured the imagination of researchers). Again, only single-centre trials were conducted, and the results were contradictory. In 1986, a committee of the Institute of Medicine met in Washington to review the evidence then extant (in six parallel-comparison trials) concerning the effectiveness of vitamin E.[6] The committee concluded that the data from these prospective studies did not warrant a recommendation for the routine use of vitamin E to prevent or modify ROP. They noted that 'a multicenter clinical trial would be necessary to provide a sufficiently large study population for definitive information on the efficacy of vitamin E in ROP.' But the co-operative action necessary to obtain this 'definitive information' has not yet been taken; and 45-years of frustrating uncertainty remains unresolved.

In the past few years, there has been an upsurge of interest in the 'oxygen paradox' (the mechanism of post-hypoxic re-oxygenation injury by oxygen free-radicals) to explain the pathogenesis of ROP and several other neonatal disorders.[7] And there is interest in ways and means of increasing the relatively poor antioxidant defences of prematurely-born infants.[8] For example, Sullivan has pointed to the low iron-binding-capacity in these neonates (and the resultant elevated concentrations of ionic iron capable of catalysing the formation of toxic oxygen free-radicals), as the deficit which may explain why they are so prone to damage by oxygen. He has urged that the preventive effect of parenteral human apotransferrin in premature infants susceptible to ROP should be subjected to formal study.[9] No one has acted on this approach; one that might shed light on a long-standing and most intriguing question: Why do most infants who develop ROP improve spontaneously?

In 1986, encouraging initial results of the use of an antioxidant (d-penicillamine) were confirmed in a randomised trial conducted in a single centre in Hungary.[10] Once more, no effort has been made to organise an independent multicentre trial to find out whether or not the favourable results with penicillamine can be replicated. And the uncertainty about the use of this approach remains unresolved.

More recently, two incidental associations were found in trials in which ROP was not the primary outcome of interest: in a trial of vitamin A supplementation,[11] and in a trial of inositol infusions,[12] ROP was less severe in infants allotted to receive the treatment under test. These encouraging observations need to be replicated by others, because they have raised hopes, again, about the possibility of finding an effective intervention to prevent all risk of ROP-blindness. If, however, the past history of proposals to eliminate this horrendous complication of premature birth is any guide, it will take years before sufficient evidence has been collected to provide reliable estimates of the effect-size of each of these plausible-but-incompletely-tested interventions.

For half-a-century the experience with ROP has demonstrated, over and over again, how difficult it is to determine the relationship between cause and effect in medicine when the course of a disorder is usually benign. As noted above, the majority of prematurely-born infants who develop the early changes of the unique retinopathy do *not* progress to blindness (among 4099 very small infants closely examined in the largest study of the natural history of ROP ever conducted,[13] 2699 developed some stage of ROP; of these only 245 progressed to 'threshold disease' that made them eligible for consideration of cryotherapy, e.g. a level of severity at which the risk of blindness was predicted to approach 50%—a risk rate that was confirmed in the outcomes of untreated eyes at age $3\frac{1}{2}$ years[14]). These features of the disorder make it manda-tory that all claims of benefit must pass the toughest tests that can be devised.

Recent reports of the unprecedented survival of extremely immature infants,[15] who are at the greatest risk for ROP, should serve as a reminder that co-ordinated, large-scale, continuous campaigns to evaluate promising interventions are long overdue. The uncoordinated, episodic, piecemeal skirmishes, that have characterised the battle to combat ROP blindness until now, are completely inadequate responses to the devastation caused by the disorder. Pocock[16] recognised the weakness as a general problem in medicine. 'Until a greater effort is made to achieve larger numbers [of patients] in ... clinical trials,' he warned, 'much published clinical research remains essentially futile, since it lacks the resources to answer the clinical questions being posed.'

(1997)

In the natural history inception cohort of CRYO-ROP (the large-scale multicentre trial of cryotherapy, noted above), 4099 infants weighing less than 1.25 kg at birth were examined systematically for signs of the retinopathy. These carefully standardised observations provided an opportunity to explore the association of long-suspected risk factors with retinal outcome.[1] The most provocative finding was a relatively low frequency of ROP among black infants (209 of 1584 = 13% prethreshold or threshold ROP) compared with their white counterparts (441 of 2158 = 20%). The discrepancy could not be accounted for by differences in the rates of retinal vascular maturation, differences in birth weight or gestational age, differences in the frequencies of small-for-gestational-age infants, differences in the medical condition or care received, nor by differences in the ophthalmologist's ability to identify the retinal changes in the eyes of infants in the two groups.

The CRYO-ROP researchers were left with the possibility that differences in ocular pigment might account for the apparent discrepancy in susceptibility. 'If retinal light exposure is a risk factor,' they speculated, greater absorption of 'incident light could explain the reduced risk we observed in black infants.' Needless to say, this has rekindled the debate about the role of exposure to light in ROP; these arguments have waxed and waned since Terry posed the question more than fifty years ago. Controlled trials to evaluate the protective effect of reducing early exposure to light have been too small and too weak to provide a convincing answer to the questions posed. Only two trials (one in 1952,[2] the latest in 1994[3]) used valid experimental design, and results in both failed to support suspicions about the harmful effect of light. At this late date, it is not very useful to pose the question in hypothesis-testing form: Does light exposure increase the risk of ROP? It is much more important to obtain a practical estimate of a purported effect-size: What is the *magnitude* of the effect of light-exposure on the risk of ROP? As the majority of susceptible infants with early retinal changes, spontaneously improve while exposed to 'normal' lighting in modern units, any increase in risk is likely to be quite small. Thus, only a very large multicentre trial (CRYO-ROP is an obvious model) can be definitive: here Pocock's warning about the perfidy of small trials could not be more timely!

If there are any doubts about the need to improve our understanding about ROP, they should be dispelled by a recent (rough) survey in schools for the blind in 23 emerging countries throughout the world.[4] Standardised examinations, made by nine ophthalmologists, led them to the conclusion that 'ROP is becoming a major cause of potentially preventable blindness among children in middle-income countries that have introduced neonatal intensive-care services for preterm and low-birthweight babies.'

33

Resolution of insoluble dilemmas

(1995)

A man was crossing a river with his wife and his mother when a giraffe appeared on the bank. When he raised his gun to shoot, the giraffe said that if he shot, his mother would die; if he didn't, his wife would die. What would you do if you were in his place?

Attributed to the Popo tribe of Dahomey[1]

'Dilemma tales', like the one quoted above, turn up frequently in African folklore. These clever and popular puzzles serve not only to sharpen the wits of tribe members, they also emphasise that in human affairs there are, very often, questions with no 'right' answers. There are only difficult choices that call up conflicting moral values.

Predicaments in the dramas enacted at the birth of marginally-viable newborn infants sometimes resemble those described in the folk tales. For example, a dynamic approach to the management of newly-born fetal infants is now one of the commonly accepted canons in the practice of present day neonatal medicine.[2] According to this belief, strengthened with the arrival of surfactant treatment, every neonate born around 23–25 or more weeks of gestation 'must be given the benefit of the doubt' with an opportunity for extrauterine life.[3] Consequently, invasive cardio-pulmonary resuscitation in the delivery room is carried out for even the smallest and most malformed babies. Immediate rescue, neonatologists argue, buys the time needed to assess the infants's status in the detail made possible by modern diagnostic techniques in the special-care baby unit. And this unhurried approach, it is held, allows the treatment team to develop a consensus about the advisability of continuing life-prolonging treatment.[4] (Another justification—one not openly discussed—is the training opportunity afforded by resuscitating the most difficult cases. One budding young rescuer bragged that he could 'bring a peach back from the dead' with the exciting new skills he was learning.[5])

The 'positive' programme (obligatory-initial-life-support) reflects a widely-held view that a 'neutral' approach (comfort-care-only requested by some parents in borderline situations) is extremely dangerous. Inaction, it is argued, increases the risk of handicapping disability should the untreated infant survive. But where is the concrete evidence to support this frequently-expressed claim?

The presumption that there is a 'continuum of reproductive casualty' (ranging from lethal damage that results in abortion, stillbirths and neonatal deaths; to sub-lethal injury seen in survivors who exhibit neurological impairments) was proposed 40 years ago by Lilienfeld and Pasamanick.[6] An association was envisioned between 'reproductive casualty' and subsequent disability related to the degree of asphyxia incurred around the time of birth. Severe, but non-fatal asphyxia, according to this thesis, leads to major neurological damage. The more frequent occurrence of milder asphyxia, it was argued, leads to lesser damage to the developing brain; and the latter may be recognised only after a long and careful follow-up. Although the argument was plausible, supporting clinical evidence has never been strong. Indeed, one heretical view now suggests that neurological damage (for example, in the form of cerebral palsy in survivors of term pregnancies) is an unreliable marker of intrapartum asphyxia, because this mechanism does not account for most instances of CP.[7]

In the very first issue of *Paediatric and Perinatal Epidemiology*, Margaret Ounsted questioned the validity of the concept of a 'continuum of reproductive casualty.'[8] She criticised the use of retrospective analyses to establish a link between intrapartum events and long-term outcome of children. And she summarised the results of her prospective study in Oxford which examined the growth and development of children born from 1970 to 1973, to mothers with hypertension in pregnancy (most of these affected women had been enrolled in a randomised treatment trial[9]). When compared with controls, perinatal mortality rates and perinatal complications in the high-risk group were very high. And unfavourable 'environmental' factors (low socio-economic status, smoking mothers and so on) were found more frequently in the high-risk group than in controls. 'Yet, despite this multiplicity of adverse pre-, peri-, and postnatal factors,' Ounsted pointed out, 'the surviving children in the [high-risk] group did not differ from the rest in a wide range of developmental tests at age 7.5 years.' 'Our findings give no support to the idea that there is an association between perinatal mortality and morbidity and long-term developmental defect. ... Rather than a diminishing gradient of early anoxic trauma and later disability, there seems to be an "all or none" effect.' 'These [high-risk] fetuses and newborn babies either die, or survive intact,' she concluded.

These findings suggest a remarkable resilience of those compromised neonates who, by natural selection, are hardy enough to survive without heroic medical rescue. And in such survivors, Ounsted advised, it is extremely important to provide a favourable on-going postnatal environment 'in which a child can regain his lost equilibrium, and express to the full his own innate abilities.' Her analysis was reinforced by earlier conclusions of Sameroff and Chandler[10] who used the phrase 'continuum of care-taking casualty' to debunk the conventional view about the long term effects of acute perinatal events. They emphasised, instead, the critical importance of the circumstances of child rearing and that of socio-economic status on developmental outcome. Werner and her associates[11] came to the same conclusion after a longitudinal survey of the fate of 1 000 live births: ten times as many children had problems related to the effects of poor early environment, compared to the effects of perinatal stress.

There is an urgent need for updated estimates of the size of the purported risk of increased CNS damage in marginally-viable survivors who are not resuscitated aggressively. Without objective data, there is simply no way to judge claims made for the 'positive' programme, since it has never been subjected to a formal clinical trial. There are ample grounds for disagreement, since many loving parents regard the quiet death of their high-risk newborn infant as only one, and certainly not the worst, in a list of undesirable outcomes. What is seen by well-intentioned neonatologists as a humane act to give a seriously compromised neonate the benefit of the doubt, is viewed by some horrified parents as an inhumane infliction of pain and suffering in the conduct of an uncontrolled and unintelligible clinical experiment without their informed consent.

There is simply no satisfactory solution to such conflicts. Game theorists label these struggles 'zero-sum' contests—one side's gain is another's loss. But we must recognise that in the 'game' that plays itself out in the delivery room at the birth of a borderline infant, the power of the 'players' is unequal and grossly unfair. The encounter follows the rules of warfare noted by the ancient Greek historian, Thucydides:[12] 'the standard of justice depends on the equality of power to compel....and, in fact, the strong do what they have the power to do, and the weak accept what they have to accept.'

Reply by John C. Sinclair and Peter W. Fowlie:
(1995)

> If your mother and your wife are drowning
> I want to know which one you would be saving (repeat)
> As for me, I would be hanging onto my mother
> And my wife, she would have to excuse
> For I can always get another wife
> But I can never get another mother in my life
>
> Calypso[1]

Unlike the dilemma cited by Silverman, this one has a solution. One may or may not agree with the conclusion, but one does recognise the method: an explicit comparison of consequences of alternative actions and of the values placed on those consequences. Note that the analysis reflects the values of the individual who is in the position of making the decision; in identifying the preferred intervention, moreover, there is no indication that the analyst has taken into account the preferences of other players—the wife, the children, the mother—who may have important views on the subject. Note also that the analysis is not directed at the issue of identifying the most promising approaches to reducing the burden of death from drowning among wives or mothers in the population.

But what has all this to do with decisions in perinatal health care?

Silverman questions the validity of the concept of 'continuum of reproductive casualty' and recommends for consideration an opposing concept whereby natural selection serves to identify those who, given non-heroic perinatal care, are destined either to die early or to survive unscathed in the long run. In support of this latter concept, he cites evidence that intrapartum asphyxia does not account for most cases of cerebral palsy and evidence that neurodevelopment in childhood can be heavily influenced by factors other than perinatal stress—early environment, socioeconomic status and circumstances of child-rearing skills. But this kind of evidence bears on the issue of the proportion of disability and handicap in childhood that is associated with particular risk factors—the population attributable fraction; it does not provide evidence either for or against the efficacy and safety of intervening at birth by treating specific risks. Thus, while we are persuaded that most cases of disability and handicap are not associated with intrapartum asphyxia, it also can be true that effective treatment of intrapartum asphyxia can reduce the prevalence of childhood disability and handicap.

Silverman cites the work of Ounsted who found that the survivors of a high-risk birth cohort did not show a disadvantage compared with lower-risk controls when they were tested at 7.5 years; in fact, if anything, their developmental scores were higher. Ounsted interpreted these observations as evidence of an all-or-none phenomenon whereby perinatal risk factors (in this case, those associated with severe hypertension in pregnancy) resulted either in early death or intact survival. We agree that a dissociation between effects on early versus late adverse outcomes does not suggest a 'continuum' model; instead, it could indicate a model of independence (because, for example, of the fact that the causes of early death and late morbidity are different). Applying this 'independence' model to therapeutic intervention, a treatment which is effective in reducing early death would be predicted to have no direct effect on late morbidity, although the proportion of survivors with late morbidity would be reduced to the extent there are more survivors.

A more extreme model to consider, which is at the opposite pole from the continuum model, is that of competing events. A 'competing event' model proposes that a risk factor or exposure that increases the number who experience early death will decrease reciprocally the number who experience late morbidity (i.e. those who die early were destined to have late morbidity had they survived); conversely, an exposure or treatment which reduces the early adverse event rate would be predicted to increase reciprocally the late event rate. Such a model is suggested by the results of overviews of randomised trials concerning the administration and monitoring of oxygen in pre-term infants.[2,3] In these examples, the early risk of death appears to compete with the later risk of retinopathy of prematurity: the exposure group that had the higher risk of early death had the lower risk of retinopathy. (We acknowledge that the differences in early death rates were, in these examples, not statistically significant.)

We see no rationale for the assumption that any one model is generalisable. Indeed, we suspect that given the variety of possible noxious exposures—genetic, asphyxial, infectious, toxic, traumatic—no one model will have general applicability. Moreover, we would not assume that a model that describes the association between early and late events in a natural history study provides a basis for predicting the relative effects on early and late outcomes following medical intervention. We note that very large sample sizes would be needed to discriminate reliably among different models that might be fitted to perinatal and childhood medical data sets.

Thus, we view model-fitting as a weak approach to important questions concerning early and late effects of perinatal risks or perinatal health care. It is important to apply the strongest scientific methods that we have, and to ensure that the method matches the question. If we want to know the fraction of disease occurrence in childhood that is associated with a perinatal risk factor, we should carry out epidemiological surveys and compute the population attributable fraction. If we want to assess the efficacy and safety of intervening with treatment in the presence of a risk factor, we should perform randomised trials. The outcomes in such trials should include outcomes identified as important not primarily by well-meaning investigators but, more cogently, by the affected surviving children and their parents.[4,5] The more frequently that we follow the lead of Ounsted and her colleagues in incorporating late outcomes into the design and conduct of randomised trials of perinatal therapies (and we have a dearth of such information at present) the better will we be able to appreciate, in specific clinical circumstances, the true relationship between early and late treatment effects.

Reply by John Watts and Saroj Saigal:

(1995)

Although we share the same conclusion as Silverman (above), we believe that the dynamic approach does have at least some justifiable application, and also that there are more fundamental issues that have not been addressed.

King[1] has described the changing attitudes of neonatologists in the United States. The Maximin approach described by Rhoden[2] which involved subscribing to a philosophy of waiting until absolute certainty that continued treatment is futile, has given way to what has been called an 'individualised prognostic strategy' where treatment is necessarily and automatically begun, but periodically re-evaluated as more information is amassed. This approach is called the dynamic approach by Silverman. It is felt by most American neonatologists to be preferable to the alternative of a 'statistical prognostic strategy' in which policy decisions (based on outcome studies) are applied to groups of infants rather than individuals (for example, policy decisions to not ventilate or resuscitate infants below a particular birthweight).

Both King and Rhoden have pointed out that the individual prognostic strategy requires an increased acceptance of uncertainty on the part of physicians. In addition, as King points out, it requires a relationship with parents that she describes as 'transparent,' using Brody's term which he describes thus: 'essentially the transparency standard requires the physician to engage in the typical patient management thought process only to do it out loud in language understandable to the patient.' [3]

Silverman, in effect, argues that the acceptance of uncertainty and the adoption of transparency should be extended to the situation before and immediately after delivery. This argument is somewhat similar to that of Botkin,[4] although the latter would restrict this degree of parental decision making to infants less than 500 gm who are born in poor clinical condition. It is almost identical to the views expressed by the combined statement of the Canadian Pediatric Society and the Society of Obstetricians and Gynecologists of Canada,[5] which recommends that resuscitation of infants of 23 and 24 completed weeks of gestation should be consistent with the parents' wishes.

One justification for the dynamic approach is that uncertainty is considerably greater before birth than afterwards. Infants may be unexpectedly more mature or unexpectedly larger, and the dynamic approach gives such infants the benefit of the doubt. However, this problem is of decreasing importance with the widespread availability of ultrasound assessment. It does, however, remain true, particularly for some groups of mothers at very high risk of prematurity, especially the poor and ill-educated; such patients are more likely to receive little or no antenatal care, possess relatively poor health education and may have uncertain dates as a result of poor compliance in the use of oral contraception. True uncertainty about the size and maturity, therefore, may be a real justification for the dynamic approach.

In addition, there is not always the opportunity to make decisions in advance. Very early labour or delivery occurs only in a very small proportion of mothers. It is usually unexpected, unwanted and tragic. Sudden crises such as this may generate a response of guilt, denial or anger, however skilled and available antenatal counselling may be. No parent is happy to make the decision to lose their infant and not a few find themselves, through no fault of their own or their physician, unable to make such a decision. Therefore, when delivery is totally unexpected and rapid, or when parents feel unwilling to make an antenatal decision the dynamic approach may remain appropriate.

Silverman gives a second quasi-justification for the dynamic approach which is that of the educational value of aggressive resuscitation. We have, frankly, never come across such a justification either overtly or covertly, and find the phraseology of the resident quoted by him equally repugnant. The final justification for automatic resuscitation is the claim that inaction runs the risk of producing an increased degree of handicap in some infants who survive despite the absence of resuscitation. Lilienfeld proposed a continuum of reproductive casualty ranging from lethality (stillbirth and neonatal death) to cerebral palsy and epilepsy in survivors; this was originally postulated as a conceptual framework for research.[6] Ounsted argued, on the basis of a study of outcomes of hypertensive pregnancies between 1970 and 1973, that there was, in fact, no continuum but an 'all-or-nothing' phenomenon.[7] However, at the time of this study premature infants in the UK were resuscitated much less frequently, and ventilators were used less often and with less success, if at all. Ounsted's description of an all-or-nothing phenomenon may well be correct for that period, and the outcome of those (largely term) pregnancies. Even though there is a poor correlation between cerebral palsy and perinatal events, the presence of a continuum of effects in premature infants which can be modified by intensive care has not been disproved. Indeed, most recent reviews suggest a stable or even decreasing rate of major impairment in the face of increasing survival of the very premature infant,[8] suggesting that aggressive and effective intensive care can shift the spectrum of morbidity to the less severe end. In addition, recent evidence suggests that in infants < 2000 gm there is a predictive relationship between ultrasound evidence of perinatal brain injury and disabling cerebral palsy.[9] Is the outcome of infants of 23–25 weeks an 'all-or-nothing' phenomenon? Withholding intensive care in these truly immature infants usually results in death. Occasionally, however, it does not—but the likelihood of such unexpected survival is unknown. In the absence of accurate information we are, indeed, left with a dilemma like those of the Popo tribe, but a dilemma which not only has no right answer, but no wrong answer either.

A further problem is that, although we have information on the impact on families of survival—wanted or unwanted—in an atmosphere of a dynamic approach, we know very little about the impact on families of the death of an infant as a selected option—and even less about the impact of unexpected survival after such choices.

Why, therefore, should we press the point that parents should be given discretion in determining resuscitation policy at very early gestation? Firstly, we can now usually be reasonably sure of size and gestation. Secondly, and more important, the outcome of interest for both parents and paediatricians is more than death. In order for very low birthweight infants to survive, they must undergo four or more months of NICU existence, some of which will be recognisably severely distressful. Indeed, in the case of the impaired survivors a very high proportion of this early existence may represent profound suffering. For some babies and parents we believe this is too high a price to pay. Such parents should be given the opportunity to make a transparently informed decision. Those parents who do not have such an opportunity or feel unwilling to make such a decision may be justifiably treated by the dynamic approach.

However, this leaves us with an issue which we find extremely troublesome and which is not addressed by Silverman. At what point is it appropriate to stop giving parents this degree of discretion? Clearly society, as represented by the courts, requires parents to take responsibility for the well-being of their infant. This includes medical care, and failure to provide it risks penalty as well as the loss of the child. Where is—and, more important, who determines—the boundary between parental autonomy and infant protection (beneficence)?

We are helped in some respects by the original 'Baby Doe' decision. This set a very clear boundary, and in neither Canada nor in the United States would the courts countenance withholding life saving surgery (and presumably intensive care) on the basis of future intellectual challenge alone. This, unfortunately, does not help us make decisions with the very low birthweight infant. Botkin[4] has suggested that where there is credible professional opinion on both sides of the question of resuscitation or intensive care the parents should have the prerogative of choice. Further, he suggests that the spectrum of parental influences should be strongest when the chances of survival are least. In conversation with at least one extremely knowledgeable parent (Helen Harrison, personal communication) it was suggested that the 50–50 point, that is 50% survival, 50% death, represented an appropriate cut-off. However, this suggestion does not incorporate the distress and suffering of survivors, an issue which we have earlier argued to be important.

Clearly, we have not found an answer to this question. We believe that approaches to the answers are not to be found through the courts nor through the beliefs and values of neonatologists or other health care professionals. Instead, the answer to policy questions, just as the answers to individual patient's questions, should be sought from parents,[10] those who have undergone the experience of an infant in the intensive care unit and even from graduates of intensive care themselves.[11]

34

'Fixing' human reproduction (1996)

Human institutions are so imperfect by their nature that in order to destroy them it is almost always enough to extend their underlying ideas to the extreme.

Alexis de Tocqueville

There is a disturbing similarity between the eugenics movement that ended more than half a century ago (1866–ca 1930), and the modern never-say-die undertaking in antenatal/neonatal medicine (1965–present). The canonical drive of eugenicists to limit the propagation of 'undesirable' offspring resembles—at the opposite pole—the fervent drive of perinatologists and neonatologists to remove all limits in the rescue of marginally-viable offspring. Both campaigns have employed extreme measures to impose intentional human design onto the imperceptibly slow, nonrandom, natural selection process for the evolutionary adaptation of our species to changing environmental conditions.

One of the first suggestions in modern times that the human race could be improved by judicious breeding was made in America, in 1848, by John Humphrey Noyes, a preacher in the Oneida Community (a utopian religious society of "Perfectionists" in central New York State).[1] Following the presentation of Darwin and Wallace's joint paper on a theory of evolution to the Linnaean Society in 1858,[2] interest in human perfectibility quickened. Although Darwin was reluctant to discuss the issue, his cousin, Francis Galton (a brilliant polymath), began to speculate about the implications of the new theory for human development. In 1865, he said,[1] 'If a twentieth part of the cost and pains were spent in measures for the improvement of the human race that is spent on the improvement of the breed of horses and cattle, what a galaxy of geniuses might we not create.'

In 1883, Galton coined the word 'eugenics' (from the Greek 'good in birth' or 'noble in lineage').[3] He defined the new field of interest as the science of improving human stock 'by giving the more suitable races or

strains of blood a better chance of prevailing speedily over the less suitable.' 'The processes of evolution,' he said, 'are in constant and ponderous
activity towards the bad and some towards the good. Our part is to watch
for opportunities to intervene by checking the former and giving free play
to the latter.'

Galton assumed that most human attributes were inherited: these
ranged from desirable traits, like talent and high intelligence, to undesirable characteristics, like pauperism, alcoholism, prostitution, criminality,
insanity, and all types of low intelligence. The social import of the evolutionary theory and its applicability to the solution of social problems were
also supported by others in Britain, notably Karl Pearson, R.A. Fisher,
John Maynard Keynes, J.B.S. Haldane, Bernard Shaw and Havelock Ellis.
Soon, organizations devoted to the dissemination of eugenic ideas for
social action were established throughout the world (e.g. America,
Britain, Germany, Scandinavia, Italy, Austria, France, Japan, and in
South America[1]).

Although Britain gave Darwin to the world, America gave his theory
an unusually quick and sympathetic reception. It has been noted[4] that
Darwin was made an honorary member of the American Philosophical
Society in 1869, ten years before his own university, Cambridge, awarded
him an honorary degree. Hofstadter pointed out that the British philosopher, Herbert Spencer, who made extensive efforts to obtain general
acceptance of the social implications of evolutionary theory, was far more
popular in America than he was at home. The 'rugged individualist,'
invoked in Spencer's interpretation of human evolution, fit the image
many Americans saw in their own society.[1]

The eugenic societies established in the US in the late nineteenth
century were short-lived; perhaps because so little was known about the
mechanism of inheritance. In 1900, when Mendel's classic paper, written
in 1866, was rediscovered, the science of genetics began to grow rapidly,
and interest in eugenics also increased. Charles Davenport, a prominent
American geneticist, persuaded the Carnegie Foundation in 1904 to
establish and support the Cold Spring Harbor Laboratories in New York
for the study of human evolution.[3] The Cold Spring Harbor site became
the national headquarters of the American Eugenics Record Office. (A
Eugenics Society was established in Britain in 1907.) In 1904, Davenport
expressed the outlook of the American eugenics movement when he
wrote:[1] 'Society must protect itself; as it claims the right to deprive the
murderer of his life, so also it may annihilate the hideous serpent of
hopelessly vicious protoplasm.'

From 1905 to the early 1930s, eugenicists in the US pursued a two-
part plan of action:[1] (1) 'negative eugenics' was focused on efforts to
eliminate detrimental traits by discouraging 'unworthy' persons from
bearing children (the 'negative' measures included marriage restriction,
sexual sterilization, and permanent institutionalization of 'defectives'),

(2) 'positive eugenics' attempted to increase desired traits by encouraging the 'better classes' to bear more children (the difficulties in carrying out the 'positive' plan in a liberal democratic society were insurmountable; action was limited to broadcasting that 'worthy' parents should have more children). For about three-decades the eugenics movement was not only a social campaign, it also became a moral crusade—a secular religion. American eugenicists spoke[1] of 'the religion of evolution,' 'the duty of upbuilding the human race,' and 'the moral implication in the doctrine of evolution.'

The 'negative eugenics' procedure of sexual sterilization for 'undesirable' people, was used frequently in the US. It has been estimated[3] that about 9000 persons classified as 'feeble-minded,' were sterilized between 1907 and 1928. In 1927, Oliver Wendell Holmes, the famous US Supreme Court Justice, handed down an oft-cited judgement.[5] It sanctioned salpingectomy for Carrie Buck, an 18 year-old 'feeble-minded woman in the State Colony [for the "Feeble-minded" in Virginia] ... the daughter of a feeble-minded mother in the same institution, and mother of a illegitimate feeble-minded child.' Justice Holmes expressed the prevailing American view of the time, when he wrote, 'It would be better for all the world, if instead of waiting to execute degenerate offspring for crime, or to let them starve for their imbecility, society can prevent those who are manifestly unfit from continuing their kind. The principle that sustains compulsory vaccination is broad enough to cover cutting the Fallopian tubes. Three generations of imbeciles are enough.'

The eugenicists racial views ('the Negro race is biologically inferior to the Mongoloid race, which in turn is inferior to the Caucasian race ... and there is a three-tiered classification of the white race, ascending from Mediterranians, to Alpines, and culminating in the superior Nordic race'[1]) became a murderous science in the hands of the National Socialists in Germany. In 1933, Hitler's cabinet drafted a Eugenic Sterilization Law that led first to atrocities by doctors, and then to 'ethnic cleansing' on an unprecedented scale of depravity and horror. The revulsion against these evil fruits of eugenics resulted in repudiation of the corrupted science by sane societies.

It is, of course, foolish to *equate* the murderous end-consequences of the eugenics movement with the results of modern efforts to preserve the lives of marginally-viable infants. In fact, the modern rescue efforts might be seen as the ultimate refutation of the ill-considered and ill-fated efforts to create superior human beings. But it is foolhardy to ignore the fact that the rescue movement is, like the eugenic programme, a myopic effort to improve on nature by increasing the 'efficiency' of human reproduction. As in all species, human reproduction is a very extravagant process. Biological flaws are so frequent that only about 20 per cent of human embryonic beings, created at conception, complete gestational development,[6,7] and neonatal losses caused by developmental errors have always been large. The zeal of rescuers, who are making unlimited efforts to 'fix' this profligacy, is impressive. But what is the price of this major uncoupling our species from natural selection? Those who remember the disconnect of knowledge from value in the eugenics debacle want to cry out (as Cromwell did in his letter to the General Assembly of the Kirk of Scotland on the third of August, 1650): 'I beseech you, in the bowels of Christ, think it possible you may be mistaken!'

(1997)

A long-forgotten story of a intense public debate about withholding life-prolonging treatment from impaired new-borns, was rediscovered recently by Martin Pernick, an American historian.[1] He found that the controversy began in 1915, after Doctor Harry Haiselden, a Chicago surgeon, refused to perform corrective surgery for imperforate anus in an infant born with numerous other non-lethal anomalies; the infant died 5-days later. Haiselden used this incident to publicise his views about allowing 'defective' babies to die. Pernick reported that Haiselden displayed dying infants to reporters, posed for newsreels cameras, delivered public lectures, and wrote a series of newspaper articles 'to rally support for his campaign against the treatment of defective new-borns.' Editorials for and against this position, appeared in newspapers throughout the US. Pernick discovered that Helen Keller, the celebrated advocate for the disabled, and the Catholic Cardinal of Baltimore were among Haiselden's most surprising supporters. Parents of handicapped children wrote pleading letters to Heiselden asking for his help in allowing their children to die. A number of official investigations of the incident involving the original infant were launched, and despite demands for the maverick doctor's indictment by the Attorney General of Illinois, the State's Attorney refused to file criminal charges. He ruled that parents had a right to withhold their consent.

In collaboration with a muckraking journalist, Haiselden wrote, and played the starring role, in a motion picture entitled *The Black Stork*. The plot of the film, Pernick found, was based loosely on the incident involving Haiselden's original patient. In the movie, the 'fictional' doctor refuses to perform corrective surgery and thereby save a severely disabled infant's life . The 'mother is torn with uncertainty,' Pernick recounts, 'until God reveals a lengthy vision of the child's future filled with pain, madness, and crime.' When the mother's doubts are resolved, she accepts the doctor's judgement, 'and the baby's soul leaps into the arms of a waiting Jesus.'

The debate raged in the US for two years, Pernick noted, but 'after 1917 Haiselden and his cause rapidly dropped from public view.' Curiously, the melodramatic movie, '*The Black Stork*' (re-titled '*Are You Fit to Marry?*'

after 1918) 'continued to be shown in small theatres and in travelling road shows, perhaps as late as 1942.'

The two-year period of national debate, early in the century, presaged the much longer 'Baby Doe' controversy in the US that erupted in the 1980s, and the dispute about elective comfort-care-only continues to the present-day (pp. 24–25). Then, as now, Pernick pointed out, the issue of withholding medical treatment becomes enmeshed with the role of the media—always eager to report an especially lurid instance of errancy. For many of Haiselden's critics, the refusal-to-treat question itself, was less troubling than his much-too-public efforts to disclose the arcane process of medical decision making. The profession's craving for 'aesthetic censorship' (Pernick's term), leads to cycles of public awareness of many ethical issues in medicine. The shifts, he concluded, 'may be related more to changes in media coverage [than] to changes in medical practice.'

35

Justice defined as fairness
(1996)

Human domination over nature is quite simply an illusion, a passing fancy by a naive species. It is an illusion that has cost us much, ensnared us in our own designs, given us a few boasts to make about our courage and genius, but all the same it is an illusion.

Donald Worster[1]

At the turn of the century, Budin taught that even when ideal environmental conditions and expert nursing care were provided for newly-born premature infants, there seemed to be a natural limit to viability (p. 75). In the opening comments of his famous lectures on the care of premature infants,[2] he said, 'We shall not discuss infants of less than 1000 grams [at birth] ... they are seldom saved, and only very rarely shall I need to allude to them.' Aggressive measures taken to breach this limit began in earnest during the 1970s; and by the 1980s, the new limit appeared to be lowered to ca 750 grams birthweight (ca 26 weeks gestation).[3] The arrival of prophylactic surfactant in the last few years seems to have driven the limit of viability even lower (p. 140).

For example, a recent report of outcomes in a case series at John Hopkins Hospital in the US (under a newly adopted policy of resuscitation and routine administration of surfactant for 142 infants born at 22 to 25 weeks' gestation—birthweight 465–975 grams) suggests that the limit of viability may now be ca 23–24 weeks.[4] The gradation of poor outcomes (severe abnormalities on cranial ultrasonography and early infant mortality) was correlated with decreasing gestational age. This led the authors to the conclusion that aggressive resuscitation and all-out treatment is indicated for infants born at 25 weeks, is questionable at 23–24 weeks, and is not indicated for infants born at or before 22 weeks of gestation. An editorial commenting on the report,[5] endorsed these recommendations, and noted the agreement with a Canadian statement concerning the management of the extremely low gestation infant.[6]

It is curious to see these efforts to promote a uniform practice for aggressive resuscitation based on the value judgements of the policy makers. This comes at a time of increasing awareness of the need to defer to the values and preferences of individual patients or their surrogates in all uncertain clinical situations. As argued repeatedly above, judgements about the advisability of aggressive treatment of marginally-viable infants are suspended in thin air when they are made without objective evidence about the outcomes of alternative courses of action (*concurrent comparison of aggressive resuscitation vs comfort care*, when outcomes-of-interest are defined by parents).

Arguments in a very perceptive analysis of present-day medical decision-making by Lynn and De Grazia,[7] are relevant to the debate about a uniform policy for the rescue of marginally-viable neonates. They describe two approaches: the traditional method, which is labeled a 'fix-it' model; and a proposed plan, which envisions an 'outcomes' model for medical decision-making.

In the modern era, they note, a mechanistic conception has guided medical action: deviations from normal physiological function are identified and then 'fixed' by specific interventions. Physicians working within this model seek objective measures of success; restoration of normal function, improved function, or prolongation of life are, for example, easily measured outcomes of 'hard fact.' ('Soft indicators' such as 'reduced pain and suffering,' 'patient's satisfaction,' 'improved well-being,' 'family stability,' and the like are avoided because they are difficult to measure reliably.) The goal of the 'fix-it' model is to standardise decision-making. Doctors present their patients with a recommendation for the 'best' course of action; patients are then free to accept or reject the advice. The ideal patient, in this model of decision-making, is one who accepts the proffered recommendation and complies with all further orders. 'Seldom does the doctor [find it necessary to present] a series of alternative possible treatments,' Lidz and Meisel have written,[8] '[because] it does not seem to the doctor to be a decision-making process but simply a question of persuading the patient to accept proper treatment.'

For example, under the 'fix-it' view of neonatal medicine's goal, when insufficient pulmonary surfactant was identified as a major defect limiting the viability of prematurely-born infants, installation of this lung-stabilizing substance became a rational intervention to rescue marginally-viable neonates. The Johns Hopkins Hospital investigators have written that 'obstetricians and neonatologists consulted with each other and with the families about the timing and the mode of delivery and the care of the [extremely premature] infant in the delivery room.' The report, however, gives no indication that 'comfort care' was offered to the parents as an alternative option to aggressive treatment given during the period under study. And there is no mention of whether or not an infant's pain and suffering, and long-term social outcomes of critical interest to the parents were taken into account each time individual decisions were made for all-out rescue.

Lynn and DeGrazia argue that the 'fix-it' model of decision-making works well when illness is acute and normal function can be restored quickly. But the approach is flawed when a medical problem is chronic and complex, and when available interventions are, at best, partially effective. They propose a decision-making model focused on outcomes judged from the patient's own perspective. 'What matters to the patient,' they point out, 'and what should matter to the practitioner, is the future possibilities that might be effectuated for [the individual] patient.' Since people in a free and plural society differ substantially in how they assess the various elements of their likely futures, uniform decision rules for life-prolonging interventions are manifestly unjust. 'We celebrate our pluralism,' Lynn and DeGrazia write, 'and are much more concerned that we defend each person's right to be different in such personal matters [rather than a concern] that any one person's views are justified, coherent, or consonant with some moral authority.' The argument is particularly timely because irreconcilable religious, philosophical and moral doctrines, plus communication barriers in a cacophony of different languages are now permanent features of all liberal democratic societies. Moreover, this heterogeneity will not disappear. John Rawls, the noted American philosopher, affirms that pluralism is the normal and inevitable outcome of free human reason over time. 'We need to recognise, he writes,[9] 'that free institutions encourage the development of differing, often conflicting, views of what constitutes a good life.'

In the hectic atmosphere of the delivery room when a marginally-viable infant is delivered, a specified definition of the limit of viability and a uniform policy for aggressive resuscitation do create a rational order. But a distinction needs to be drawn in this situation between a 'rational decision' in the 'fix-it' model, and the 'reasonable choice' in the 'outcomes-oriented' approach. The difference follows Rawls argument: The concept of reasonableness is an element in a society that sees itself organised as a system of fair cooperation, a system that tolerates wide differences in values and preferences. Rationality, on the other hand, is concerned only with a search for the most effective means to a narrowly-defined end. Justice, defined as fairness, Rawls concludes, rejects the idea that the 'reasonable' can be derived from the 'rational.'

The rescue principle in medicine holds to the view that the prolongation of life is paramount among all goods; everything, from this perspective, must be sacrificed for it. But no sane society, Ronald Dworkin points out,[10] would try to fulfill that ideal, any more than a sane person would organise his/her life according to the extreme terms of the rescue principle. 'Modern medicine has created so many vastly expensive forms of medical [treatment],' Dworkin argues, 'it would be preposterous that a community should treat longer life as a good that it must provide at any cost—even one that would make the lives of its people barely worth living.' Similarly, each family must be allowed to make these agonizing decisions for themselves. 'The most important feature of Western political culture,' Dworkin writes,[11] 'is a belief in individual human dignity. People have a moral right and the moral responsibility to confront the most fundamental questions about the meaning and value of their own lives for themselves.'

(1997)

After 4 years of comprehensive study, the Institute of Medicine's Committee on Care at the End of Life in the US, recently issued[1] a scathing rebuke of the medical profession for inattention to end-of-life care. 'Medical culture,' the panel charged, '... tolerates and even rewards the misapplication of life-sustaining technologies while slighting the prevention and relief of suffering. Humane care for those approaching death is a social obligation from those directly involved,' the report has declared.

A number of obstructions have interfered with fulfilment of the responsibility. Not the least of these is lack of training; and that deficit, an editorialist recently noted,[2] begins in medical school. A survey of medical schools in the US revealed 'only six of 126 schools required a course on death and dying ...'.[3] The IOM panel also focused on the medical schools' neglect: 'Dying is too important a part of life to be left to one or two required (but poorly attended) lectures.'

Full recognition of the extent of pain and suffering during the prolonged dying of neonates kept alive by rescue machinery is long overdue. The issue is certainly paramount in the minds of parents.[4] Perhaps recent awareness of the long-neglected topic of pain in neonates (pp. 106–10) will bring about a much-needed change in teaching about death and dying in these mute patients. We need to understand what Jeremy Bentham intuited about the treatment of animals. 'The question is not,' he once said, 'Can they reason?, nor Can they talk?; but Can they suffer?'

36

'Methods-based' reviews
(1996)

When the ordinary modes of practice have been attempted
without success, it is for the public good ... that new remedies
and new methods of chirurgical treatment should be devised.
No such trials [of these innovations] should be instituted,
without a previous consultation of other physicians and surgeons, according to the nature of the case.

Thomas Percival[1]

Thomas Percival (1740–1804), a pre-eminent physician in Manchester,
was asked to act as referee in a number of serious controversies that took
place among his colleagues late in the eighteenth-century. These experiences led him to draft a Code of Institutes and Precepts in 1794 to guide
the 'professional conduct' of doctors. With the above-quoted exception,
his Code focused more on medical etiquette (e.g. matters of fees, con-
sultations, seniority among colleagues, and so on), than on moral issues
that turn up in doctors' everyday encounters with patients. Faden and
Beauchamp have pointed out[2] that Percival used the behaviour expected
of a 'Christian gentleman' as his model for a standard of professional
decorum. The Codes were published in book form in 1803, one year
before he died. The influence of Percival's *Medical Ethics* lasted for many
years after his death; the book was widely acknowledged as the most
authoritative reference on the subject throughout Britain and the US.
Many of his sentences and paragraphs were copied verbatim in subsequent ethical principles in medicine drawn up in the nineteenth century.

Curiously, Percival's admonition about a doctor's obligation to consult
peers before using a previously untried treatment was not reiterated.
As Levine has noted,[3] no similar caution was published for more than
150 years. For example, the revulsion against the barbaric experiments carried out by Nazi doctors led to the adoption of the Nuremberg
Code in 1949:[4] It stressed that human experiments 'should be so designed
... that the anticipated results will justify the performance of the

experiment.' But there was no mention of how this value judgement should be made—there was no statement about a need for peer review of experimental plans. Ladimer, in 1963,[5] appears to be the first, in the modern era, to suggest that protocols for human research be submitted to a review group for prior evaluation. But the Declaration of Helsinki, published the following year,[6] made no mention of this pre-condition. Finally, in 1975, when the Helsinki Declaration was amended in Tokyo,[7] committee review was formally adopted as a requirement (Principle 1.2):

> The design and performance of each experimental procedure involving human subjects should be ... transmitted to a specially appointed independent committee for consideration, comment and guidance.

The review committee was envisioned as an advisory, rather than a regulatory body. Enforcement of the provision was to take place at the time of publication; journal editors were seen as the *de facto* regulators (Principle 1.8):

> Reports of experiments not in accordance with the principles laid down in this Declaration should not be accepted for publication.'

In the past quarter-century, prospective peer review of each research proposal involving human beings, has been required in most developed countries. Review boards, usually in individual institutions (often called 'IRBs'), must make independent determinations:[8] (1) of the rights and welfare of research subjects, (2) of the appropriateness of methods used to obtain informed consent, and (3) of the risks and potential benefits of the investigation. However, from the very beginning of mandatory peer review, the credibility of IRBs was, and continues to be questioned.

For example, Levine has charged that the boards can create the appearance of protection of research subjects ('a record that will warm the cockles of any bureaucrat's heart'), but these appearances are, too often, deceptive. IRBs spend so much time on trivial changes in the wording of the consent forms, he observes, there is little time left to consider the details of negotiations with patients to obtain that consent; and there is little or no oversight of actual performance.

Initially, membership in IRBs was limited to immediate peers (clinicians and basic scientists); lawyers, clergy and lay persons were conspicuous by their absence, or, at most, by token appointments. Later, representation in the committees was broadened to reflect community interests, but this did not silence the critics. McNeill has written[9] that experts have a 'unique commitment to research that favours the interests of science ... and deliberation often slights the concerns of patients.' Additionally, he suggests, there is a conflict of interest in the IRB system: Each institution stands to gain from the research it conducts. 'It must be

assumed,' he declares, 'there is pressure on research ethics committees . . .
to approve research, and [thereby] attract funding and kudos to their
[own] institutions.' And the economic pressures are enormous when, as
happens increasingly, staff members must generate their own salaries
from funds awarded for research. The result, McNeill concludes, is a
system for 'allowing research on human subjects with a minimum of
interference.' Annas' criticism is similarly harsh:[10] 'IRBs as currently con-
stituted do not protect research subjects but rather protect the institution
and the institution's investigators.'

From the very outset of the institution-based reviews, it has been obvious that individual interpretations of regulations have varied widely.
The inconsistencies were revealed most clearly in multi-centre studies.
For instance, in 1979, Kavanaugh and coworkers[11] submitted a protocol
(for a survey of genetic counselling services) to IRBs in 51 institutions
in the US. It took an entire year to obtain final authorisation: 11 IRBs
decided a review was unnecessary, 28 approved the protocol as submitted, and 12 approved after one or more modifications were made.
More than 15 years later, the discrepancies in judgement are, if anything,
even more conspicuous. Alberti comments[12] that [in Britain] 'this has led
to a progressively larger groundswell of complaint from research workers
frustrated at the delays incurred, the costs involved, and the unnecessary
duplication of effort.' It might help, Foster advises,[13] if all IRBs would
focus on the same fundamental questions: 'Does the project ask an important question? Will the study design allow that question to be answered?
Are the risks to research subjects acceptable? Will the autonomy of the
subjects be respected by their consent being obtained?'

The question about study design deserves particular emphasis.
Commonly, IRBs spend little or no time examining methodological rigour
in each proposal, on the assumption that a critical review of 'Method' will
be conducted later by experts in a funding agency. But design is basic:
it needs to be appraised before any other aspect of a proposal is even
considered. If a study design is so flawed that it cannot possibly generate
reproducible observations, it is by definition unethical and should be dis-
allowed without further consideration. Rutstein once wrote,[14] 'When a
study is in itself scientifically invalid, all other ethical considerations
become irrelevant. There is no point in obtaining 'informed consent' to
perform a useless study.' A strong case can be made for requiring that
the size and methodological strategy of each study proposal be examined
initially by an independent biostatistician (with no ties to the applicant's
institution). Under this plan, *only* those protocols certified as authentic
tests of the specific questions posed in research protocols, would be
submitted for IRB reviews.

The most convincing indication of the need for change is found in the
numerous studies of the quality of published medical studies cited
recently by Altman.[15] In a commentary entitled 'The scandal of poor

medical research,' he charged that 'huge sums of money are spent annually on research that is seriously flawed through the use of inappropriate design, unrepresentative samples, small samples, incorrect methods of analysis, and faulty interpretation.' Since this plethora of methodological errors was detected easily after publication, it affirms that the current system for prior review is simply not weeding out proposals that should not be implemented.

This disturbing state of affairs was predicted accurately by Prescott, two decades ago.[16] He warned then that unless more attention is paid to improve the quality of medical research '[many investigators] will spend much of their time on work which is doomed in advance to be of no medical or scientific merit ... [and] the literature will continue to produce articles where the conclusions do not follow from the data. Worst of all, such articles will continue to be believed.'

(1997)

The most recent revision of the World Medical Association's guidelines for research involving human subjects, in 1996, added no specific provision about 'Method.'[1] As in previous guidelines, investigators are told that 'Biomedical research involving human subjects must conform to generally accepted scientific principles.' The institutional review board is, once again, viewed as an advisory, not a regulatory committee. As a result, the validity of methods used in clinical studies is still evaluated after the fact, by the peer-review process used by medical journals. Knowledgeable 'peers' function as gatekeepers, charged with the responsibility of barring the publication of improperly designed clinical studies after they have been carried out!

For example, a survey of the declared policies of 102 biomedical journals was carried out in 1995.[2] Only 48 of the reviewed journals required specific documentation of IRB approval as a prerequisite for publication. The surveyors were concerned about the role of the IRB in upholding 'ethical standards'; principally, issues related to informed consent. And they reaffirmed the conventional view: the responsibility for critical review of methodology rests with 'journal editors and their consultant staff of reviewers to ensure clinical and scientific rigor....'

Why do we continue to tolerate this myopic *post facto* system? The practice fails to protect patients from enrolling in useless studies—investigations that will be rejected later as uninterpretable because of poor study design. An Advance Review Option proposed by Weiss several years ago,[3] seems a reasonable solution (a complete description of the study, including dummy tables and figures, is submitted for publication before the study is undertaken). Moreover, the ARO plan is testable.

Patients need all the protection they can get from what Porter calls 'medicine's notoriously messy mix, the itch for knowledge and the need to act.'[4]

37

Non-replication of the replicable (1996)

Knowledge does not automatically order itself in human terms. ... More startling, and contrary to workaday beliefs of most scientists, knowledge does not even accumulate, in the simplest, additive sense.

Melvin Konner[1]

Haines and Jones[2] recently commented on the unfortunate delays in the implementation of many findings of medical research, and, they pointed out, the problem is a very old one. For example, James Lancaster demonstrated that lemon juice prevented scurvy in 1601, but 146 years elapsed before the experiment was repeated (by James Lind in 1747).[3] Another 46 years went by before the British Navy began (in 1795) to supply lemon juice for its ships at sea; and this preventive measure was not adopted by the merchant marine until 1865.

The medical literature, Haines and Jones point out, is littered with examples of research findings that have not found timely acceptance in practice. Similarly, it should be noted, many research leads requiring further critical evaluation before they are accepted as 'true,' are also left dangling in what might be called 'existential limbo.'

There are many examples of unsatisfactory closure in the evolution of modern neonatal medicine. One such episode began in Buffalo, New York, in 1960, when an association was described linking maternal bleeding during pregnancy and hyaline membrane disease (HMD) diagnosed at postmortem in prematurely-born neonates who succumbed in the first seven days of life.[4] This association and the observation that the 'membrane' itself was composed of fibrin, led to a suspicion there might be a defect in fibrinolysis in prematurely-born infants. Following this lead, the Buffalo investigators conducted a prospective survey of fibrinolytic factors in the blood and the lungs of premature infants with and without HMD:[5] the survey revealed low levels of these substances. This support for the suspicion led to a pilot study of treatment with human plasmin (activated fibrinolytic enzymes) involving 12 premature infants with severe respiratory distress. The initial observations were followed by a small randomised double-blind trial of the new treatment in 33 neonates with early clinical signs of the respiratory distress syndrome (RDS). Mortality in infants treated with urokinase-activated plasmin was lower than in affected neonates given placebo, or in others given streptokinase-activated plasmin. These preliminary results encouraged the investigators to continue the randomised trial of the effectiveness of UK-plasmin treatment until 100 infants with early RDS were enrolled; mortality in symptomatic infants allocated to the treatment arm of the trial was appreciably lower than in placebo treated controls.[6] Since UK-plasmin was difficult to prepare and unavailable for general use, the Buffalo investigators then undertook a multicentre randomised double-blind trial to evaluate a prevention strategy: plasminogen (the precursor of the fibrinolytic enzyme, plasmin) or placebo was administered to 500 low birthweight infants within the first hour of life.[7] The overall occurrence of RDS was identical in both arms of the trial; but severity and duration were diminished, and overall mortality was significantly lower in infants who received prophylactic plasminogen.

Curiously, these encouraging results in a carefully planned series of studies conducted over a period of more than 15 years and culminating in a rigourous large-scale randomised trial, were almost completely ignored (except for one uncontrolled case-series in Reims, France, describing 'considerable improvement over classical survival rates in 14 premature infants suffering from respiratory distress treated with a combination of plasminogen and urokinase'[8]). For example, after completion of the Buffalo treatment trial, the results were presented at a national conference,[9] where these investigators noted that '[Our] study must be repeated in larger numbers and by other investigators.' The proposal was met by a haughty put down: 'It would take an extraordinary effort,' one prominent researcher replied, 'to test a hypothesis for which I see little support.' This disinterest turned out to be typical. The provocative findings in the very large prevention trial failed to ignite a flicker of response from the neonatology establishment. The results of years of work in Buffalo were quickly forgotten.

Another intriguing lead in the management of prematurely-born infants—also completely ignored—surfaced in Hungary in 1973, when a group of investigators began to use d-penicillamine (DAP) in the treatment of neonatal hyperbilirubinemia (based on the chelating action of DAP, which inhibits heme degradation in newborn animals). When a very low incidence of retinopathy of prematurity (ROP) was found in the infants so treated for jaundice, the Hungarian group began to use DAP to prevent the retinal disorder (now based on the knowledge that DAP is an antioxidant, and that it inhibits collagen synthesis, this treatment might, the researchers reasoned, decrease vitreal proliferation in ROP p. 137). The results in observational studies were encouraging;[10]

and, in 1986, a randomised clinical trial of the effectiveness of DAP was carried out. Among 204 infants enrolled in the trial, no ROP (greater than Grade II) was seen among 71 survivors in the treatment arm of the trial; 6 infants developed ROP (greater than Grade II) among 70 survivors in the control group, and 4 of these progressed to Grade III or more.[11] No independent efforts were made by others to repeat this trial.

In a recent letter to the editor,[12] the Hungarian investigators reported that over a 19-year period they have treated approximately 20,000 term and preterm neonates with DAP to prevent severe jaundice and ROP. No adverse effects or late complications of treatment were found in systematic follow-up of survivors.

What accounts for the reluctance to repeat the work of others? The aloof behaviour is a sad comment on the value system of medicine as it struggles to become scientific (e.g. the encouraging shift now taking place from authority-based to 'evidence-based medicine'[13]). Innovators are highly valued, and, justly celebrated because of their 'originality;' unfortunately, replicators are not held in high esteem, and their work is denigrated because it is 'imitative.' But this outlook is a misinterpretation of what the scientific enterprise is all about: 'organized scepticism' is the cornerstone of modern science. Doubters are not only required, they have an obligation to *act*. And their actions—attempts to repeat the clinical experiment—are not made to affirm the original claim, but to probe the limits of its applicability. Without sceptics who are willing to undertake the crucial work of replication, progress in scientific medicine falters and becomes haphazard.

As has been argued above, repeatedly, there is no way to know when our observations about complex events in nature are complete. Our knowledge is finite, Karl Popper emphasised, but our ignorance is infinite. In medicine, we can never be certain about the consequences of our interventions, we can only narrow the area of uncertainty. This admission is not as pessimistic as it sounds; claims that resist repeated energetic challenges, often turn out to be quite reliable. Such 'working truths' are the building blocks for the reasonably solid structures that support our everyday actions at the bedside.

(1997)

When a statistical approach was first taken up by agricultural scientists, to guide field research, the methods were cumbersome. Large numbers of observations over prolonged periods of time were needed to provide reliable estimates of the frequency of chance variations. In the early 1920s, when R.A. Fisher began to work on these problems, he became aware of the practical difficulties, and he explored the mathematical implications of using small numbers of observations in trials to measure the effectiveness of manure in increasing crop yields. Fisher's solution was brilliant:[1] plots of land were subdivided into blocks, and within each block, manure-treated and untreated strips were arranged in *random* order. The new approach freed researchers from the previous stringency of large sample size, and a test could be concluded in a single growing season. Fisher's methods for small-sample-size problems were revolutionary; his experimental designs were adopted in many fields of applied research throughout the world.

However, Fisher advised caution about accepting the results of a single experiment.[2] 'In order to assert that a natural phenomenon is experimentally demonstrated,' he warned, ' we need, not an isolated record, but a reliable method of procedure ... we may say that a phenomenon is experimentally demonstrable when we know how to conduct an experiment which will rarely fail to give us a statistically significant result.' A similar warning was sounded early in the history of clinical trials by Donald Mainland, an American biostatistician.[3] 'The only way to learn something about the safety of our numerical findings,' he noted, 'is by more extensive exploration under other conditions, in other places, and at other times.'

There is an obvious collision here: the deeply held convictions of methodologists (who call for independent replications of randomised clinical trials, RCTs) collide with the equally strong beliefs of moralists (who condemn any RCT carried out after the superiority of a treatment has been demonstrated in one previous trial). There is simply no way of reconciling these opposing views, and it would be foolhardy to force a rigid rule-based resolution. On the other hand, it might be useful to set out a few principles to guide a middle course that would balance the interests of present and future patients.

'Rules dictate results, come what may.' Dworkin asserts.[4] 'Principles do not work that way; they incline a decision one way but not conclusively, and permit a judgement that fits the situation. Principles allow us to think.'

38

Who defines 'futility'?
(1997)

> We need to recover a religious sense that death is not an evil
> ... that outlook might save us from the triumphalist tempta-
> tion to slash and suture our way to eternal life.
>
> Paul Ramsey[1]

Parents have always recognised and feared the brutal truth about human
reproduction: It is, as in all species, a very wasteful and imperfect
process. 'Parents often tell me,' Edmund Hey has written,[2] 'that they
dread severe handicap in a young child more than death itself. In addition they often fear that medical and nursing staff will not recognise
and respect these feelings.' But something new seems to have taken place
on the other side of the Atlantic. A surprising number of American
parents now seem to be demanding the very kind of heroic neonatal
rescue so widely feared in the past!

For example, several years ago a report revealed[3] that doctors in the
US refused a mother's request for aggressive life-support of her severely
damaged child, identified as Baby L. The doctors argued that active
rescue would prolong suffering needlessly and would, therefore, be inhumane. The provocative case report triggered a response from the editor
of the *Journal of Perinatology*.[4] He asked neonatologists on the editorial
board to give their individual views about the 'refuse-to-treat' issue in
the US; that is to say, the clash between claims of parental autonomy
and physicians' sworn obligation 'to do good (commit acts) and avoid
harm (omit acts).' The neonatologists acknowledged that unreasonable requests for prolongation of life were coming up with increasing
frequency. Most on the editorial board asserted that parents cannot
compel doctors to inflict needless pain and suffering; but they gave
no indication that this view was, in fact, guiding everyday practice.
For example, one editorialist surveyed the attitudes of 61 neonatologists
and learned that 82% thought a ventilator should not be offered to a
(hypothetical) 21-week-gestation, liveborn infant weighing less than
500 grams. Despite these beliefs, 62% of the same respondents said
they would ventilate the infant if the family said, 'Do all you can.'

More recently, Fleischman also observed[5] that overtreatment of neonates is increasing in the US. Families are requesting continued aggressive treatment, he pointed out, for infants who are much too damaged to
receive any benefit from intervention. Phoon recently wrote:[6] 'In a single
month I have witnessed several children with severe disease ... whose
parents in nearly every case wanted aggressive treatment. ... [After]
discussing the potential complications of prematurity with expectant
mothers at 21 to 24 weeks gestation, most ... wanted "everything done."
Indeed, rarely has a parent requested withdrawal of support for severely
ill neonates. ...'

What are the underlying dynamics of these unrealistic requests? King
has suggested[7] that a communication problem may, on occasion, account
for the disturbing phenomenon. Unjustified optimism may develop, she
points out, when a marginally-viable baby seems to do well in the first
day or so after birth, and then begins to fail. As the doctors become
increasingly convinced by the accumulation of findings that indicate a
worsening prognosis, a time gap may develop between the understanding of the caregivers and that of the parents. When the implications of
technical information collected during the progressive decline are not
fully explained to parents, they cling to hopes that become increasingly
unreal.

However, it is hard to believe that a time/information gap is the chief
reason for these misperceptions. As noted above (p. 63), the uncom-
promising views of the right-to-life movement and those of organisations
of the disabled erupted and were widely publicised in the US at the time
of the 'Baby Doe' affair in the 1980s. That publicity had, and continues to
have, an influence in forming the unrealistic 'never-say-die' mind-set
of some new parents in that country. And, it must also be recognised,
the idea that everything is possible has been an essential part of the
American dream for a very long time. Alexis de Tocqueville noticed this
when he studied American institutions early in the nineteenth century.
He said,[8] 'Nowhere does [the American] see any limit placed by nature to
human endeavor; in his eyes something that does not exist is just something that has not been tried.'

In the 1980s, the American 'gung-ho' spirit was celebrated in breathless
news accounts about the achievements in neonatal medicine. These
dramas were not enacted in isolation; they took place in the context of
widespread excitement about all medical explorations ballyhooed in print
and broadcast media. For example, there was a continuous flow of reports
describing miracles achieved with organ transplantation and artificial
heart implants. Two American sociologists, Renee Fox and Judith Swazey,
longtime participant-observers in that field, have written[9] a very perceptive account of what they termed 'experiments perilous' conducted in the
US in the 1980s when efforts were made to implant the Jarvick-7 artificial
heart. They were troubled by what they saw as a 'courage to fail' value

system adopted by the artificial organ innovators. 'This ethos,' they explained, 'includes a classically American frontier outlook: heroic, pioneering, adventurous, optimistic, and determined. But it also involves,' they added, 'a bellicose, "death is the enemy" perspective; a rescue oriented and often zealous determination to maintain life at any cost; and a relentless, hubris-ridden refusal to accept limits.' Fox and Swazey were increasingly disturbed to see how the 'courage to fail' outlook was subjecting vulnerable patients to excruciating distress. Additionally, they observed, the field of organ replacement has 'epitomized . . . our pervasive reluctance to accept the limits to the biological and human condition imposed by the aging process and our ultimate mortality. . . .'

Use of the possessive pronoun 'our,' acknowledges that the all-out-rescue mentality is no longer an isolated state of mind confined to the rescuers. It has been so oversold, some gullible patients and their families simply refuse to face the impossible. An example of the bizarre situation was recorded recently by Annas[10] in a report of the management of 'Baby K'—an anencephalic infant—in the State of Virginia. The diagnosis was made prenatally and the mother refused to accept the obstetrician and a neonatologist's advice to terminate the pregnancy. At birth, the doomed infant was placed on a respirator and ventilated at the mother's insistence (the father played no role in the drama). The doctors urged that the ventilator be discontinued because it served no humane or medical purpose; but the mother insisted on continued life-support. They turned to the hospital's ethics committee for a decision, but it failed to come to grips with the dilemma—the committee advised that a legal solution be sought to the impasse. The mother finally agreed to allow infant to be transferred to a nursing home on condition that the hospital would readmit 'Baby K' if respiratory symptoms worsened; and the infant did return on two occasions. The hospital then sought a ruling in the courts, arguing that it was not obliged to provide 'inappropriate' medical treatment; but the plea was rebuffed. A trial court ruled that 'absent a finding of neglect or abuse, parents have the right to make decisions about medical treatment for their children.' An appellate decision also favored the mother's stand, and added, 'It is beyond the limits of the court's judicial function to address the moral or ethical propriety of providing . . . treatment for anencephalic infants.'

Annas reported[11] that the unfortunate 'Baby K' was still in a nursing home; and, assuming the diagnosis is correct, 'she may be the longest-lived anencephalic infant in medical history [age 1-year and 4-months, as of February 1994].'

The compliance of doctors who, at the insistence of parents, prescribe treatments they know to be futile, and the refusal of the courts to support the advice of other doctors who wish to resist such unreasonable demands, are disturbing developments. They suggest that medicine is seen, increasingly, as a vendible good. As Annas observed,[11] many physicians and hospitals in the US appear to 'treat medicine as a business in which medical services are provided on the basis of the patients' desires rather than medical indications. It is becoming more and more difficult for physicians to refuse whatever patients and their families demand.' If this continues, he predicted, gloomily, 'medicine will be seen as a consumer commodity like breakfast cereal and toothpaste.'

Reply by Amnon Goldworth and William E. Benitz:

(1997)

Silverman explores the vexing question why 'A surprising number of American parents now seem to be demanding the very kind of heroic neonatal rescue so widely feared in the past.' We agree with his claim that 'the all-out-rescue mentality' of physicians has caused parents to demand treatment even where the success of any medical intervention approached zero. But there is a related issue concerning physicians' willingness to comply with the unrealistic demands of parents.

Silverman provides one reason which is based on 'refusal of the courts to support the advice of ... doctors who wish to resist such unreasonable demands. ...' But there are several other reasons that are suggested by the discussion of the Baby L case.[1,2] In that instance, the consensus among the medical care team (including the chiefs of service, the primary care physicians, the hospital counsel and the ethics committee) was not supported by other physicians, as reported in the *Journal of Perinatology.*[3]

There are three distinct reasons why disagreements occurred. First, some physicians questioned or challenged the position of others that the child's best interests would be served by further life-preserving treatments. We believe that this serves to illustrate the fact that judgements about the best interests of patients derives from assessments about the benefits and burdens of treatment. But, purely technical assessments do not exhaust the meanings of 'benefit' and 'burden.' What is included are subjective perspectives generated by the values of the physician. The second reason concerns the ambiguous nature of the concept of futility. Unless a treatment is physiologically so futile that the probability of successful treatment is zero, differences in the value of treatment outcomes, whatever the probability of success in achieving those outcomes, can lead to conflict. The ambiguous nature of the concept of futility underlies the mother's insistence that treatment of her anencephalic infant, 'Baby K', be continued. (The baby lived for another year beyond February 1994.) The third reason is the lack of understanding of those processes by which decisions can be made without provoking conflicts between physician and parent. Silverman touches on this problem in presenting King's suggestion that a failure in communication may generate unjustified optimism about treatment success in parents. But the heart of the problem has to do with a failure to define a process by which decisions can be reached between physician and parent which avoids conflict.

It is our belief that any combination of these three reasons, as reinforced by the rescue mentality referred to by Silverman, leads physicians to capitulate to the unreasonable demands of parents.

39

Fitting targets to holes
(1997)

It ain't what a man don't know as makes him a fool, but what
he does know as ain't so.

Josh Billings (1818–1885)

Daniel Boorstin has commented[1] on the breathtaking cosmological
models that have been put forward, based on the postulate that 'the
entire universe we observe, and unimaginably far beyond, was created
out of a single tiny vacuum fluctuation having zero energy content at
an incredibly early time ... our universe was, quite literally created out
of nothing. These amazingly bold conjectures about the entire universe
and our place in it,' Boorstin writes, 'are the consequence of the application of developed technology to the processes of scientific discovery and
the rise of the mechanised observer.'

One of the important implications of the enormous expansion of scientific information is the transformed relation of data to meaning. 'Before
the age of the mechanised observer,' Boorstin observes, 'there was a
tendency for meaning to outrun data. The modern tendency is quite the
contrary, as we see data outrun meaning.'

An early example of the glut of data in medicine took place in the
mid-19th century, soon after Karl August Wunderlich introduced routine
measurement of body temperature in the care of patients.[2] The large
amount of data generated by the thermometer created much dissatis-
faction among practitioners. 'With its unavoidable escort of millions of
facts,' one physician observed, 'and with the diagrams whose curves
would compete with waves of the ocean, clinical thermometry makes
upon the mind of the practitioner first an impression of awe, and second,
one of disappointment.'

A more recent example of an instance when data outdistanced meaning, began in the 1950s, just as the modern revolution in perinatal medicine was getting under way. The US National Institute of Neurological
Disease and Blindness (NINDB) launched a large observational study
which was to involve a prospective cohort of 50 000 pregnant women

and their subsequent offspring born in twelve large medical centres in that country. The aim of this huge effort was to obtain information about 'all possible' antecedents of cerebral palsy and other neurological disorders in early childhood. 'The paucity of strong hypotheses concerning the factors contributing to [these conditions],' the planners noted, 'necessitated a study design of large scope and wide range.'[3] The plan, entitled 'The Collaborative Project on Cerebral Palsy, Mental Retardation and Other Neurological Disorders of Infancy and Childhood (later shortened, mercifully, to 'The Collaborative Perinatal Project' [CPP]) called for the collection of a pooled set of data in a uniform manner by trained teams of obstetricians, paediatricians and neurologists—the 'mechanised observers' (to use Boorstin's term). Patient enrolment began in 1957; and the enormous amount of data collected quickly overwhelmed the capacity of the NINDB staff assigned to analyse it.

The CPP Study was severely criticised at a meeting on research methodology in 1963 (at which time the major data processing problems had been ironed out, and almost 33 000 of the projected 50 000 pregnant women had been enrolled).[4] The critics pointed out that the planners had not set out specific hypotheses *before* the data were collected. It was revealed that there had been difficulties in deciding which predictor variables should be included. As a result of the varied interests and the large number of consultants and participants involved in these decisions, the variables multiplied: '... for every page that was excluded, two pages were added.' In the end, 162 predictor variables were chosen, and each case generated 'several thousand bits of information.' One critic observed that '... multiple variables [are] being substituted for the judgement required in identifying fruitful research questions ... I believe too little attention has been given to identifying questions of special interest and to making sure that the quality of the data required for these special questions is adequate.'

Additionally, questions were raised about the selection bias in the recruitment of the study population. It turned out that the enrolees were not a representative sample of the US and did not even reflect the ethnic composition of the cities in which the collaborating centres were located.

At the time of these critical comments, US$33 255 000 had already been spent on the CPP Study over the six-year period from 1957 to 1963. Despite the lambasting and constructive suggestions for change, the study lumbered on unchanged, and an additional 20 000 pregnant women were enrolled. By the end of 1978, 22 years after enrolment began, a grand total of US$122 004 000 had been expended on this mammoth undertaking (T. Matthews, personal communication, 1979) and the end was not yet in sight: It was estimated that an additional US$1 051 000 would be required in 1979. (The unwillingness of the investigators to change in response to the criticism of the methodologically flawed study after 1963, reminds one of the 'crackpot realist' who throws away a million dollars, arguing that 'you can't just junk a project into which we've already sunk a hundred thousand dollars.')

The penchant for collecting a large number of 'mechanised observations' unrelated to explicitly-worded prior hypotheses set down in the study protocol, did not end after the clear lessons taught by the CPP Study. Unfortunately, the compulsive practice in the conduct of many clinical studies, including randomised trials, continues; and it adds enormously to costs (to say nothing about the interpretative problems when the mass of data are then dredged using computer programs to look for 'statistically significant,' but unpredicted associations). Peto and his colleagues are blunt in their advice about this pernicious problem:[5] 'Most [clinical] trials would be of much greater scientific value if they collected ten times less data, both at entry and during follow-up, and were, therefore much larger.' And Jolley uses a wonderfully vivid image to illustrate the danger of *post hoc* reasoning:[6] 'The "Texas sharpshooter" fires a shot randomly into the side of a barn, then draws a target centered on the hole. Dredging data for "significant" p values fits targets to holes.'

(1997)

Viewed in retrospect, the collection of massive amounts of 'mechanised information' in the notorious cerebral palsy project (above), and the even more immense collection of 'mechanised observations' obtained in routine electronic fetal monitoring, seem quixotic. In 1996, MacDonald charged[1] that 'Despite the "intensive obstetrics" of the past 25 years ... the frequency of cerebral palsy remains unchanged at about 2 cases per 1000 term infants.'

Interest in the antecedents of cerebral palsy has now shifted from the prolonged preoccupation with intrapartum asphyxia, to a new focus on antenatal events long before delivery. (The geographically based case–control studies in Western Australia have indicated that 'intrapartum asphyxia is a rare cause of cerebral palsy.'[2]) The pathophysiology, of what is now termed 'hypoxic-ischaemic cerebral injury,' has been described in fascinating detail, and optimists now expect that highly-specific therapies will be available soon. Perlman has warned[3] that these exciting treatments 'carry with them the potential for major side effects.' The need for large-scale randomised trials of the new approaches could hardly be more obvious.

40

Medical 'manners' on trial
(1997)

The real greatness of a nation, its true civilization, is measured by the extent, in this land, of obedience to the unenforceable.

Lord Moulton

Shortly before his death in 1924, John Fletcher Moulton, a Lord Justice of appeal, gave an impromptu speech at the Authors' Club in London. A reporter made a verbatim record of the talk and it was published posthumously in *The Atlantic Monthly* under the title 'Law and Manners.'[1] In his comments, Moulton defined the three great domains of human action: positive law, 'manners,' and free choice.

The realm of positive law, he observed, is designated in official statutes that must be obeyed. (Kidder noted[2] that this jurisdiction might have been labeled 'obedience to the enforceable,' since there is an expectation that all transgressions will be punished.) At the opposite end of the scale, Moulton defined a realm that includes all actions in which 'we claim and enjoy complete freedom.' While the scope of action in the latter may be smaller than the positive law, he asserted, certain freedoms of choice (e.g. religion, mode of life, selection of a mate, etc.) are very highly prized in most developed societies. Between these areas, Moulton said,

> lies a large and important domain in which there rules neither positive law nor absolute freedom. In that domain there is no law which inexorably determines our course of action, and yet we feel that we are not free to choose as we would.... It grades from a consciousness of duty nearly as strong as positive law, to a feeling that the matter is all but a question of personal choice.... [It] is the domain of obedience to the unenforceable. That obedience is the obedience of a man to that which he cannot be forced to obey. He is the enforcer of the law upon himself.'

This thoughtful classification, formulated more than seventy-years ago, may provide a revealing map of the territories of current and future medical actions. As the power of interventions has increased, the moral strength of medicine may come to lie in its 'professional manners:' the extent of self-restraint for the common good exercised by individual practitioners—the size of the middle ethical domain described by Moulton.

For example, a new device for the treatment of failing hearts was approved recently as 'safe and effective' by the US Food and Drug Administration. Bray reported[3] that this 24-ounce implantable pump was developed, at a cost of about US$ 25 million, to keep cardiac patients alive while they wait for a transplant. The cost of the new pump itself will be US$ 45 000; with the surgical procedure to install the device, the cost will increase to US$ 110 000; and the price of each eventual cardiac transplantation will be an additional US$ 72 000. These huge expenses do not include the surgeons' fees, other doctors' bills, immunosuppressive drugs, and so on.

According to the US Food and Drug Administration, 15 000 to 20 000 patients become potential candidates for heart transplantation in America each year. Bray noted that the list of patients who request the procedure keeps growing (the number on the waiting list in 1993 was 6 269, a growth of 71% over the previous four-year period). On the other hand, there is a shortage of donors (2 300 hearts were available for transplantation in 1993, an increase of only 35% over the previous four years). Since many patients die while waiting for rescue, the new pump is envisioned as a 'bridge to transplant.' As a consequence, the heart shortage in the US will intensify: more very sick patients will be able to stay alive longer than in the past. (While the new device was under test, one patient was kept alive for 17 months with this mechanical assistance.)

Use of the pump will make it possible for large numbers of patients whose overall medical status is extremely poor to receive transplants. Since the sickest patients receive the highest priority for this form of rescue, the costs for the care of these patients with serious and complex disorders will be higher, and the clinical course will be less favorable than in the past. Inevitably, individual doctors caring for patients dying of heart disease will be under enormous pressure to use the effective new 'bridge to transplant.' The struggle has become increasingly familiar in present-day medicine: there is a conflict between private choice and the common good.

The American bioethicist, Daniel Callahan points out[4] that when his field of study was inventing itself in the 1960s, it lost sight of two significant issues. First, he faults modern bioethics for its failure to examine, with sufficient imagination, the idea of the public interest, as opposed to that of the moral uses of individual choice. Second, the tendency of bioethicists to 'reduce the problem of the common good to justice, and the individual moral life to the gaining of autonomy,' Callahan writes, '[has] left a moral void.' The early focus on personal autonomy came about in the 1960s when a number of reports revealed a pattern of abuse of the rights of patients who were used as research subjects without their knowledge or consent.[5] The revelations led to the development of what Callahan calls *regulatory ethics*. For example, the establishment of the Institutional Review Board (IRB) system in 1966 was the first concrete accomplishment of the emerging field of bioethics: it provides evidence of the early preoccupation with individual rights.

Callahan calls attention to the relatively unnoticed but 'potent way in which biomedical innovation and [medical practices] were shaping the background culture in which individual decisions would be made.' The culture was exerting a powerful influence on individual decision. 'Even as autonomy was being enthroned,' he emphasises, 'its content and context were being manipulated by a tacit background culture as powerful as it was invisible.' The above noted example of cardiac transplantation is a dramatic demonstration of how a biomedical development has changed individual perspectives, and that of social institutions. As discussed here previously (pp. 168–69), the way we have come to think about ourselves and our lives has been profoundly affected by the availability of transplantation; it has fostered a 'spare parts' mentality.[6] The soon-to-come 'bridge to transplant' promises further to intensify change and confusion about how we think about the natural limit of human life. And yet, as Callahan asserts, 'It is remarkable how little reflection there has been within bioethics on the meaning, import, and acceptability of [such] changes for the way we live our lives.'

Callahan calls for the development of a '*cultural bioethics*, to serve as a counterpoint and counterweight to the reigning regulatory bioethics.' And, he suggests, a 'communitarian bioethics would want to begin an analysis of the way in which culture shapes individual choices by creating the context and limits of these choices.' The nightmare-like prospect of a huge gap between supply and demand brought on by the 'bridge to transplant' pump may, very shortly, bring the field of cardiac transplantation face to face with one of Callahan's questions about the adoption of every new medical intervention: 'What kind of culture will we be engendering by the pattern of private decisions that eventually emerges from the need to make decisions?'

Modern medicine's civility will be tested significantly; and not so much by what doctors do, as by the extent of individual practitioners' self-restraint for the common good. As Moulton might have put it, their 'manners' will be on trial.

(1997)

Since 1994, Bray notes in an updated report,[1] that three models of ventricular-assist pumps have been approved in the US by the FDA for use as 'bridges to heart transplantation.' Not surprisingly, the gap between supply and demand has persisted. The United Network for Organ Sharing reported (in 1994, the most recent year for which there was complete data in the US) 6 378 patients awaited heart transplants, but only 2 340 received them.

Nonetheless, heart transplant centres have proliferated all over the US, Bray finds, and an alarmed Health Care Financing Administration has now urged restraint. But the technology has spread rapidly: Medicare (which pays hospitals and physicians for medical care of persons over 65 years of age) spent nearly US$ 45 million for 494 heart transplants in 1995. 'Heart transplantation [in the US] is not ready for greater demand,' Bray explains, but his words of alarm seem to be falling on deaf ears .

41

Sanction of whose beliefs and values?
(1997)

In so far as ethics provides a sound guide to living, it must have life's own attributes: its pliability, its adaptiveness, its sensitiveness to the occasion.

Lewis Mumford[1]

The explicit requirement of *informed* consent for treatment, as noted here previously (pp. 72–84), is a relatively new condition imposed on the traditional relationship between doctor and patient. The transition from the older and simpler rule to the first instances in which the issue of informed consent was established in case law, took place in the US courts during the 1950s.[2]

The Supreme Court of North Carolina ruled, in 1955, that the failure to explain the risks involved in surgery 'may be considered a mistake on the part of the surgeon.' Two years later, in *Salgo v. Leland Stanford Jr. University,* the California Court of Appeals was the first to add the word 'informed' when it described a doctor's affirmative duty to reveal 'any facts which are necessary to form the basis of an intelligent consent by the patient to proposed treatment.' Only after this disclosure, the *Salgo* court ruled, may a doctor ask for a patient's written permission. It was the latter landmark decision, legal scholars have said, that created the expression 'informed consent:' it proclaimed the new responsibility of doctors. The following year the Supreme Court of Minnesota reinforced the affirmative duty of disclosure. The court held a doctor liable for not telling a patient, before surgery, about alternative forms of treatment that would not have exposed the patient to risks associated with the operative procedure that was, in fact, performed.

The concept and the requirement of informed consent were ultimately adopted in the codes of medical conduct by most Western countries in the 1960s and '70s. But the arrival of the doctrine was not welcomed by everyone—many observers were, and remain to this day, openly sceptical about the truthfulness of the consent ritual in everyday settings. Studies of the disparity between pronouncement and practice were reviewed by Katz.[3] He noted that informed consent in medicine has the quality of a fairy tale. Nothing has changed the historical practice of minimal disclosure, Katz opined, because informed consent has never really taken hold beyond the *pro forma* exercise of obtaining a patient's signature on a consent form.

Now, after almost 40 years of experience with the requirement, Robert Veatch, a highly respected American bioethicist, has made a startling proposal:[4] *Abandon* informed consent! Interestingly, his radical advice is not based on the well-known problem of deviations from the ideal. Veatch's charge is fundamental: Clinicians are unable to obtain valid consent to treatment, he argues, because they are incapable of guessing which treatment option will serve a particular patient's best interests.

A review of the rocky history of the informed-consent dogma makes it clear, Veatch notes, that the physician is still expected (as in the days before the requirement was enshrined) 'to determine what is "medically indicated," the "treatment of choice," or what in the "clinical judgement" of the practitioner is best for the patient.' This pattern of medical decision-making no longer makes sense, he suggests, because 'it rests on the outdated presumptions that the clinician's moral responsibility is to do what is best for the patient ... and that there is some hope that [a doctor] can determine what is the patient's best interest.'

The 'best interest standard' has become implausible, Veatch declares, because judgements about the 'best' option are now recognised to be entirely subjective. And, since we tolerate a reasonable range of discretion in all areas of human decision-making under conditions of uncertainty, 'it makes sense to replace the best-interest standard with a "standard of reasonableness" ...' Studies of the current philosophic theories of the concept of 'the good' lead to a radical conclusion. Veatch writes: 'There is no reason that a physician or any other expert in only one component of [the numerous organic, psychological, social, legal, occupational, religious, aesthetic, and other elements that comprise total] well-being should be able to determine what constitutes the good for another being.' Moreover, it is 'understandable that specialists should overvalue the benefits of their field,' he continues; 'they not only make the values trade-offs atypically, they also make the moral trade offs atypically.'

There is some empirical evidence that supports Veatch's fears that doctors may use their own scale of values when they make decisions 'in the patient's best interest.' For instance, Schneiderman and coworkers asked,[5] 'Do physicians' own preferences for life-sustaining treatments influence their perceptions of patients' preferences?' They surveyed the responses of 104 patients with life-threatening illnesses who were asked to indicate their preferences for four hypothetical courses of action (ranging from heroic to minimal interventions). And they compared the patients' choices with the replies of 24 physicians (each was responsible for the care of one or more of the surveyed patients).

The doctors were asked to respond in two contexts: first, to predict what their individual patients' choices would be; and then, the doctor's personal choice (i.e. if the doctor was to find him/her self to be in the same clinical state as the patient). There was poor correspondence between the patients' choice for self and the physicians' predictions of their patients' choices. Disturbingly, the doctors' predictions corresponded more closely with the choice physicians would make for themselves. These observations are consistent with the suspicion that led to the survey: doctors are not always able to understand their patients' preferences for life-prolonging treatments.

The disunity described in this survey will, very likely, increase. Englehardt has emphasised[6] that Western societies are becoming explicity and stridently pluralistic. The recognition of a pluralism of views regarding the good life, he notes, suggests that 'custodians of the moral order in the next century will ... be like good bureaucrats who follow procedures respecting the freedom of a nation's citizens without imposing a particular view of the good life.'

If, as Veatch suggests, informed consent cannot assure that the increasingly wide variety of patients' beliefs and values will shape decisions in medicine, what, then, are the alternatives? Although he makes a number of interesting proposals, Veatch's declaration needs to be heard widely, and preeminently, because of the difficult *questions* he poses. Note, in this regard, when a man tells a waitress that he has been served a rotten egg, the complainer is not obliged to lay a fresh one in its place.

(1997)

A nation-wide Canadian survey of doctors and other health care workers in intensive care units has revealed a disturbing disjunction in attitudes concerning withdrawal of life-support from critically ill patients.[1] When asked to rate the importance of each of 17 determinants to be considered for this drastic step (e.g. likelihood of surviving the current episode of illness, patient's advance directives, premorbid cognitive function, likelihood of long-term survival, etc.), there was close agreement in the responses of 1 361 health care personnel (ICU physicians, nurses, and house staff).

The respondents were then presented with contrived, but realistic scenarios of critically-ill patients, and asked to choose one of five levels of care (ranging from comfort care to full aggressive management). Now the responses varied widely, and specified characteristics of the respondents (gender, age, time since graduation and ICU experience) associated with each choice were also highly variable. 'The results indicate,' the researchers concluded, 'that factors idiosyncratic to the health care providers are major determinants of decisions to withdraw care.' These findings were consistent with other studies cited by the Canadian authors, and the accumulated body of empirical data suggested (see p. 181) 'we must recognise that even when clinicians make decisions based on the best evidence available, their own ethical, moral, and religious values influence their medical decision making.'

As noted earlier (p. 157), a lawyer and professor of philosophy have reviewed[2] a similar, but more ambitious study—the Study to Understand Prognosis and Preferences for Outcomes and Risks of Treatment, known as SUPPORT—that enrolled a large cohort of patients with life-threatening illness (ca 50% risk of immanent death) in five US teaching hospitals.[3] The researchers spent two years surveying the circumstances of gravely ill patients admitted to ICUs in these hospitals, and they isolated several disturbing features of care given to dying patients. In the second two-year period of study, a parallel-management trial was carried out, in which patients and their physicians were randomised by the doctor's speciality group to receive either a resource-rich intervention or usual medical management. 'Bluntly put,' the reviewers wrote, 'the intervention failed. In none of five areas identified as special problems by the study's first phase did the intervention achieve any improvement that was at all substantial or unambiguous.'

Many explanations for the disappointing results were put forward, but 'the most eye-catching outcome of the SUPPORT study,' the reviewers concluded, will surely be the failure of its attempt to ameliorate what has been identified as some of the worst features of death in the hospital.' The verdict of George Annas, an American attorney and ethicist, was more plain-spoken.[4] 'If dying patients want to retain some control over their dying process,' he said, 'they must get out of the hospital if they are in and stay out of the hospital if they are out.'

42

Mindless existence
(1997)

There is no good reason why a person who might have died quickly and easily in an earlier era should now have to die a worse death or remain alive much longer under degrading circumstances. Why should we have to accept this kind of medical progress?

Daniel Callahan[1]

In 1993, an infant girl with hydrocephalus, meningomyelocele and deformed lower limbs, was born in the Netherlands.[2] The attending physician decided there was no treatment that could keep her alive for more than a few overwhelmingly painful months. On the third day of life (after consulting several specialists, and after obtaining the approval of the parents), the doctor administered a sedative followed by a curare-like drug. The infant died in her mother's arms 15 minutes later. The doctor was arraigned on a criminal charge, but a District Court refused to punish him. The judge ruled that the doctor acted to spare the girl from a life of unbearable, incurable pain. News commentators noted that the legal decision, made in April 1995, was bound to stretch the limits of the relatively permissive policy for euthanasia already in place in the Netherlands.

Technically, euthanasia is illegal in Holland.[3] Under Article 293 of the Dutch Penal Code, it is clearly a criminal offence: 'He who takes the life of another person on this person's explicit and serious request will be punished with imprisonment of up to 12 years or a fine of Dfl. 100,000.' However, physicians who conform to three guidelines recognised by the courts, are not subjected to criminal sanctions. The preconditions are: (1) Voluntariness—the patient's request must be persistent, conscious and freely made); (2) Unbearable suffering—suffering cannot be relieved, and both physician and patient agree that the medical condition is beyond recovery or amelioration; and (3) Consultation—the attending doctor must consult with a colleague about the genuineness and appropriateness of the request for euthanasia. (Recently,[4] the Royal

Dutch Medical Association made an additional recommendation: Whenever possible, terminally ill patients should demonstrate their voluntary role in the act of euthanasia, by administering the fatal drug to themselves.)

The conditions have been set out[5] because euthanasia has been gaining increased public support and the co-operation of the medical profession in the Netherlands. Nation-wide surveys on a number of socio-cultural subjects were conducted in Holland on six occasions from 1966 through 1991.[6] Among other questions in a personal interview, those surveyed were asked, 'What should a doctor do when a patient asks him to end his suffering by administering a lethal injection?' In 1966, nearly half of the respondents answered that a physician should not give the injection; 4 years later, less than one-quarter gave this answer; the percentage against euthanasia continued to fall; in 1991, only 9% gave a negative response. The proportion who agreed that a lethal injection should be given on-request, rose sharply between 1966 and 1970, then increased gradually, reaching 57% in 1991. Most of the decrease among those against euthanasia was offset by an increase in the percentage of respondents who said the answer would depend on specific circumstances. Surveys in the US from 1950 through 1991, revealed a similar shift:[7] 36% of those who replied favoured euthanasia in 1950; assent increased to 63% in 1991. Public policy will change, the American authors predicted, to reflect the wishes of patients and their families to retain greater control over their own fate when life is threatened by disease. And, indeed, there have now been repeated efforts to pass 'death with dignity' laws in a number of States in the US. In 1992, a Canadian judge ruled that people have the right to demand that life-support be removed, even when they are not dying, if they find life intolerable in the circumstances in which they must live it.[8] Australia's northern territory passed an 'assisted suicide' law in 1995.

These events confirm the decline of a traditional doctrine in Western societies: a weakening of conviction about the sanctity of every human life. The erosion has caught the attention of Peter Singer, the provocative Australian philosopher who has never been shy about spelling out the full moral implications of our behaviours. He points[9] to a decision in the House of Lords as the specific moment when 'British law abandoned the idea that life itself is a benefit to the person living it, irrespective of its quality.' The decisive change came about in 1993, when the Law Lords ruled in the case of Tony Bland[10] who was caught in a human stampede on 15 April 1989. Thousands of sport fans pushed, and hundreds were crushed against a fence when they tried to get into the grounds of Hillsborough Football Stadium in Sheffield; ninety-five people died. Bland's chest was crushed and he suffered a prolonged period of asphyxia in the near-fatal incident; he was left in a persistent vegetative state as the result of severe brain damage.

Singer reports that when the attending doctor determined that Bland's state was hopeless, he decided to stop tube feedings and he notified the coroner of this plan. The coroner, who was investigating the deaths in the Hillsborough disaster, agreed that it was pointless to keep the severely damaged man alive. Nonetheless, he warned that the doctor risked criminal charges if any action was taken that would end Bland's life. The impasse was taken to the lower courts for adjudication, and, after conflicting judgements, the case finally came to the Law Lords in 1993 for a final decision. The High Court ruled that to withdraw life-support, including the discontinuation of feedings by stomach tube, was 'not only legally, but also ethically justified.' 'The utter hopelessness of ... Bland's condition,' Singer points out, 'led the judges to see that technological advances in medicine have made it impossible to retain the principle of the sanctity of human life. Instead, they switched to an ethic that sensibly takes into account whether sustaining life will benefit or harm the human being whose life is to be sustained.'

The change is momentous. (It is in direct opposition, for example, to the stand taken by right-to-life advocates at the time of the infamous 'Baby Doe' episode in the US:[11] Neonatologists were forbidden to take future quality of life into consideration when treating severely compromised neonates.) But the Bland decision in Britain does not legalise active euthanasia of the kind tolerated in the Netherlands. Instead, the Law Lords preserved the dubious distinction made in the criminal law between acts and omissions: The difference between ending a life by a deliberate act (a lethal injection) as opposed to ending that same life by withholding life-sustaining care (tube feeding). And the Lords admitted that although the distinction is difficult to defend, 'Still the law is there, and we must take it as it stands.' The ruling ended with an admission that the law has become 'morally and intellectually misshapen;' and the jurists called for new legislation. The judges could hardly have done more, Singer notes, to show clearly the need for a new approach to life and death decisions.

Ronald Dworkin, the American legal scholar, points out[12] the conviction that all human life is sacred may turn out, paradoxically, to provide a powerful argument *for*, rather than against, euthanasia. For example, some patients believe their own lives would be worse, if they were kept 'alive' in a persistent vegetative state by the full panoply of modern life-prolonging machinery. And, these patients are convinced, they are most respectful of the human contribution to the sanctity of their lives when they make plans to avoid the grim fate of a mindless existence. Forestalling death in a way that caregivers approve, when, in fact, the rescue action is a horrifying contradiction of that patient's view of the meaning of life, becomes, Dworkin asserts, 'a devastating, odious form of tyranny.'

(1997)

Hendin has recently written a highly critical review of what he terms the 'legal sanction to assisted suicide and euthanasia' in the Netherlands.[1] Among other charges, he asserts that the fall in the suicide rate in that country (from 16 per 100 000 population in 1983 to 13 in 1992) 'may well be due to the availability of euthanasia.' And, significantly, the drop in suicide has been greatest among the elderly (in those 50–59 years of age, the rate fell from a peak of 23 per 100 000 in 1982 to 15 in 1992; among those 70 years of age and over, the rate dropped from 31 in 1983 to 20 in 1992). 'In a culture accepting of euthanasia,' Hendin alleges, 'the distress [of physical illness in the aged] is seen as a good reason for dying. It is perhaps not so far-fetched to describe euthanasia as the Dutch cure for suicide,' he concludes.

Hendin also detects an increased interest in legalising euthanasia in the US. And he attributes the trend to 'fragmentation in the culture ... [the loss] of a shared set of values, leading many to believe that anything goes if it is chosen freely, regardless of social consequences.' Hendin makes a plea for 'caring beyond cure;' he points to the inequities in the US health care system, and the need to lobby for improved palliative care in terminal illness. This view is echoed by Doctor Joanne Lynn, director of George Washington University's Center to Improve Care of the Dying:[2]

> If society continues not to make caring alternatives available, but allows the option of being killed, then we must not wear blinders to what is really at stake—that is, whether this society prefers to leave dying people so bereft of hope that being killed is to be preferred to living.

The debates in the Netherlands and in the US, about social policy in the extremely controversial topic of appropriate level of care for the terminally ill, continue unabated. For example, the ministers of health and of justice in the Netherlands recently commissioned a national study of medical end-of-life decisions made for neonates and infants.[3] Physicians who attended 338 consecutive deaths (32% of the 1 041 deaths within the first year of life in 1995) were sent questionnaires; and a random sample of neonatologists, paediatric intensive-care specialists, and general paediatricians were interviewed. In more than one-half of all the events studied, an end-of-life medical decision was made prior to the time of death (these antemortem decisions were made most frequently in the neonatal intensive care units). Most of the decisions to withdraw or withhold life-sustaining treatment were made because 'there was no chance of survival, or a poor prognosis for later life;' and in some instances drugs (usually opioids) to alleviate pain and symptoms were administered 'in doses that may have shortened life.' Interviews revealed that most of these paediatricians had withdrawn or withheld treatment from a neonate at least once in their careers, and only one respondent could not conceive of a situation in which he/she would be able 'to give drugs to end life or refer patients to a colleague prepared to do so.' Parents were involved in most end-of-life decisions, the respondents reported; and decisions were never made against the parents' wishes. 'Dutch paediatricians seemed in our study to promote quality-of-life considerations as an important reason to forego life-sustaining treatment in a substantial number of [severely compromised] cases,' the researchers concluded. However, they added, 'Nearly all paediatricians believed that some form of public control on decision-making about the end of life in neonates is necessary.'

At the same time, future debate on the other side of the Atlantic will, undoubtedly, be shaped by a recent ruling of the Supreme Court in the US. There are differences, the Justices have now held, between 'the long legal tradition protecting the decision to refuse unwanted treatment ... and the right to assistance in ending one's life.'[4] But the decision has left a great deal unsaid; the Justices seem to imply that the individual States are now 'free to experiment and to make physician assisted suicide legal if they so choose.' Developments in the US during the next few years may prove to be very interesting.

43

Interventions on an unprecedented scale

(1997)

The mind of man has removed the stopper of the medicine bottle. The chemical genie formerly imprisoned within now stands before us. He is a spirit known to work miracles, but also to wreak havoc—to improve life or destroy it.

Louis Lasagna[1]

In a 1959 lecture entitled 'The Practical Uses of Theory,' Hans Jonas, a respected moral philosopher, examined[2] what he perceived to be a new relationship between theory and practice in the modern age. Over the next quarter-century until his death, Jonas reflected, wrote and lectured about the growing impact of technology on the human condition, and on the need to rethink our moral obligations. He began by looking back at traditional ethics and noted that it dealt, for the most part, with the here and now. In the past, proper conduct was visible in everyday life. The time-honoured maxims of ethical demeanour referred to current behaviours: 'Love thy neighbour as thyself'; 'Tell the truth'; 'Do unto others as you would wish them to do unto you'; and so on. The effective range of human action was small, Jonas observed, 'the time span of foresight, goal setting, and accountability was short, control of circumstances limited.' The long run of consequences was left to chance, fate, or providence. 'The short arm of human power,' he noted, 'did not call for a long arm of predictive knowledge.'

In medicine prior to World War II, for example, the remedial power of doctors was very limited. As noted above (p. 20), Lewis Thomas recalled[3] that his father, a general practitioner in semirural Connecticut during the early part this century, was influenced by Sir William Osler's teaching of *therapeutic nihilism*. The nihilists rejected most of the remedies in common use, as more likely to do harm than good: 'there are only a small number of genuinely therapeutic drugs—digitalis and morphine best of all.' When the older Thomas made home visits, the only indispensable drug in his bag was morphine; adrenaline was carried in case of anaphylactic shock, an emergency which never turned up. In due course, insulin was added to the short list.

When Lewis Thomas entered medical school in 1933, very little had changed. For example, although there had been considerable progress in understanding the causation of infectious diseases, the course of study was, if anything even more conservative than it had been thirty-years earlier. 'Its purpose,' Thomas recalled, 'was to teach the classification and recognition of disease entities ... the treatment of disease was the most minor part of the curriculum, almost left out altogether.' The medical students came to realise that 'we could do nothing to change the course of the great majority of the diseases we were so busily analysing, that medicine, for all its facade as a learned profession, was in real life a profoundly ignorant occupation.'

Needless to say, the revolutionary developments in medicine during and following World War II changed everything. And the explosive increase in technical knowledge, Jonas wrote, 'informed by an ever-deeper penetration of nature and propelled by the forces of the market and politics has enhanced human power beyond anything known or ever dreamed of before. Modern technology has introduced actions of such novel scale, objects, and consequences that the framework of former ethics cannot contain them. The duty of knowledge,' he continued, 'is now beyond anything required in the past: Now knowledge must be commensurate with the causal scale of our action.' Unfortunately, predictive knowledge always falls behind technical knowledge; and 'the gap between the ability to foretell and the power to act,' Jonas warned, 'creates a novel moral problem.'

The search for and application of new drugs to treat cardiac arrhythmias, discussed earlier (p. 49), is a modern cautionary tale that reveals virtually all of the dangers feared by Jonas. Thomas Moore has recently written a detailed and chilling account[4] of that little noticed episode; he labels it 'America's worst drug disaster.'

The story begins in 1972, Moore reports, when a large American company made a decision to diversify and enter the lucrative field of drug manufacture. A chemist in the company had just created a new compound modelled on the widely-used local anaesthetic drug, 'procaine,' and a pharmacologist suggested that the new would-be anaesthetic (subsequently labelled 'flecainide') might be useful as a suppressant for patients with irregular heartbeats. Tests in laboratory animals revealed that flecainide did indeed have potent antiarrhythmic properties. Now the long hectic race to the clinic began. Similar local-anaesthetic-like drugs ('encainide' and 'tocainide') were also under development by the company's competitors. Like flecainide, the rival compounds were categorised as Class I antiarrhythmic drugs).

Over a six-year period, studies of flecainide were conducted first, in normal volunteers, and then in cardiac patients with premature ventricular contractions (PVCs). The new agent appeared to be unusually effective in suppressing the ventricular arrhythmias; and, Moore notes, this encouraging information came at a very propitious time. In 1978, a causal link was postulated connecting PVCs (assumed to be signs of a heart's electrical instability) and the risk of sudden cardiac death. 'Any prophylactic program against sudden death,' a leading cardiologist declared, 'must involve the use of antiarrhythmic drugs to subdue [PVCs].' Some cardiologists warned against treating asymptomatic patients on the basis of this unproved 'suppression hypothesis' (there was no concrete evidence to support the hope that suppressing premature beats would prevent sudden death). Nonetheless, the claim must have seemed reasonable to many doctors, because the number of prescriptions written in the US for antiarrhythmic drugs grew phenomenally to nearly 12 million in the year 1979. Encouraged by the growing market, the company drew up a plan for the clinical development of flecainide. Moore points to a crucial stipulation in the plan: suppression of PVCs (not sudden death) was adopted as the primary outcome to test the effectiveness of flecainide. Much to their later regret, the American drug regulation authorities (FDA) concurred in this pivotal decision to choose a surrogate outcome instead of mortality as the criterion for effectiveness of all the new generation of Class I drugs then under test.

Over the next eight years, with increased use of flecainide and the similar drugs, it became clear that the new agents could suppress and at other times induce lethal cardiac arrhythmias—the drugs were thought to be implicated in a worrisome number of sudden deaths. But the companies and most doctors seemed convinced that these adverse events were rare and, in any case, were outweighed by demonstrable benefits (i.e. the suppression of PVCs). After much debate and numerous meetings within FDA and with the drug companies, approval was granted in 1986 with the requirement for a warning label calling attention to the risk of *pro*arrhythmic effects and 'reserving treatment for patients in whom benefits outweigh the risks.' The caution could not have been taken seriously, Moore opined, because two years later pharmacists were filling 57 000 prescriptions for flecainide every month—a 50 per cent increase over the previous year.

Questions about safety and effectiveness of these drugs persisted among a sceptical minority, who complained that controlled trials (as required by American law) had not been carried out before FDA approval. Belatedly, a 27-centre randomised clinical trial was mounted by the US National Heart, Lung, and Blood Institutes (NHLBI)[5] to test whether the suppression of ventricular arrhythmias with flecainide, encainide or moricizine would reduce mortality compared with controls who received a placebo. Only patients who survived a heart attack were eligible for this

Cardiac Arrhythmia Suppression Trial (CAST); additionally there had to be documented evidence of asymptomatic or mildly symptomatic ventricular arrhythmias, and a demonstration that these ectopic beats were suppressed with the drug under test before each candidate was enrolled. (It is important to note that the design of CAST called for a one-tail test of the pretrial hypothesis. The likelihood of lethal effects was thought to be too remote to require the more conservative two-tail test which would consider the probabilities of either effectiveness or *harm*.)

Recruitment was begun in June 1987 at centres in the US, Canada, and Sweden. In April 1989, CAST was truncated three-years earlier than planned, when it was found that the pretrial assumption was wrong— two of the drugs were harmful. Twice as many patients receiving flecainide or encainide died as compared with controls. As Moore points out, CAST finally provided a definitive test of the relevance of the surrogate outcome. Not only did effective suppression of PVCs fail to prevent sudden deaths, with these two drugs suppression was associated with more fatalities than in nonsuppressed controls! Patients receiving moricizine (the least effective suppressant) or placebo experienced an insignificant but favourable trend in mortality.

The CAST results caused considerable breast-beating in the FDA, but, surprisingly, the outcome was of only moderate interest to news media. Moore is appalled by the failure of reporters to probe the overall dimensions of the disaster. Approximately 200 000 patients in the US were taking flecainide and encainide. Even under the most conservative assumptions, the estimated total number of deaths comes to more than 5 000 in one year's time! Moreover, if only the excess deaths among patients receiving other Class I antiarrhythmic drugs during the two-year interval of CAST are taken into account, there must have been tens-of-thousands of drug-related fatalities in the US. The number of similar deaths in other countries has never been reckoned. The total, Moore charges, is without precedent in modern medicine.

The NHLBI-sponsored evaluation of antiarrhythmic drugs did not end in 1989; the original trial continued as CAST II with a new protocol in which only moricizine was now compared with placebo.[6] In 1990, while CAST II was still *sub judice*, moricizine was approved by the FDA, with a warning that it should be used only for 'life-threatening rhythm disturbances.' Nonetheless, the drug was advertised in medical journals as 'Now available—effective and safe [*sic*].' But the moricizine trial, CAST II, ended like its predecessor: the second trial was terminated early because of 'excess mortality' in the treatment arm. And the research team concluded (with a tortured understatement): 'CAST I and II demonstrate that suppression of ventricular arrhythmias has not been linked to improved survival.' 'In this manner,' Moore reports, 'the saga of the antiarrhythmic drugs sputtered to a quiet and inconclusive close.' Only two newspapers carried a brief story reporting the results of CAST II.

What went wrong with the laudable attempt to fashion logical treatment based on a very reasonable, but untested, hypothesis? Hans Jonas might argue that the potency of the new drugs combined with such limited predictive knowledge created an enormous burden of responsibility. And it is the magnitude of the stakes that leads to Jonas' pragmatic rule: 'give the prophecy of doom priority over the prophecy of bliss.'

An 'imperative of responsibility' might have persuaded the clinicians to use the most rigorous methodology (concurrent controls) in their *earliest* attempts to investigate a beneficent use of the untested drugs. Additionally, Jonas might have counselled a very slow and cautious acceptance of the drugs for general use. As he once warned,[7] 'the tempo [of progress], compulsive as it may become, has nothing sacred about it ... too ruthless a pursuit of scientific progress would make its most dazzling triumphs not worth having.'

44

Preoccupation with 'autonomy'
(1997)

... everything which contributes to the happiness of society,
recommends itself directly to our approbation and good-will.
Here is the principle which accounts, in great part, for the
origin of morality.

David Hume[1]

The increased capability to determine precise details about the state of
health of neonates has fostered emergence of a view that they are
patients in their own right and not the inseparable wards of their
parents. And, it is argued, emotionally distraught parents simply cannot
be expected to place the earthly existence of newly-arrived, flawed
offspring above all other family values. In keeping with this concept,
neonatologists often consider themselves the unbiased protectors of their
mute patients' best interests and assume an advocacy role. A claim is
often made that doctors are justified in overriding parents' wishes when
making controversial decisions about complex life-prolonging treatment.

However, this 'atomist' view, which sees the newborn in isolation,
needs to be challenged. It is an example of what Etzioni has called 'the
celebration of individualism that has been carried too far ... under-
cutting the legitimisation of the community and of the public realm.'[2]
Similarly, Nelson writes,[3] 'the intensity of focus on patients' interests—
considered as the interests of splendidly-isolated individuals—reflects a
kind of moral obtuseness ... we would do better to design a system of
medical decision making sensitive to a broader range of values.'

The reason atomism has had such a powerful influence, Churchill
suggests,[4] is related to its emotional appeal in depicting the self in a
seductive way. This outlook in Western cultures stresses 'an individual's
freedom, dignity, and power,' he points out, 'it portrays persons who are
free to choose social relationships and whose lives remain essentially
unchanged by such choices.' Since individual existence is essential to
human beings and social existence merely discretionary, according to

this narrow view, 'individuals constitute the moral unit of meaning.' Thus, it is claimed, 'derivative social relationships are ethically uninteresting except as they form an occasion for, or the setting of, individual choice.'

Atomistic philosophy has skewed the emphasis in bioethics, Churchill argues, as indicated by the current 'preoccupation with the concept of autonomy.' [see Callahan's similar argument, pp. 176–77]. By stretching autonomy beyond the appropriate range of its application, Churchill asserts, it has been used as 'a moral "trump card" in situations for which it is ill-suited.' This has had the effect of diminishing the importance of justice and other values; and 'it ultimately warps the principle of autonomy as well.' Churchill takes the view (derived from Hume) that 'we cannot begin with a premise of asocial individualism and arrive at a viable social ethic. The earliest experiences of humankind are social, Churchill points out: 'They involve the succour and support of family into which one is born and about which no choices are made. Affiliations and alliances are, therefore, a necessity;' he concludes, '[they are] a matter of survival throughout a person's life....' A similar Hume-like argument about the contested terrain of autonomy in bioethics has been made by Murray.[5] Although 'autonomy remains a vital moral bulwark against oppression,' Murray has suggested, 'it is not an all-encompassing guide to living good lives or building good communities.'

David Hume's explication of the origins of moral beliefs was set out in his first publication, *A Treatise of Human Nature*. The work was written in 1734 when he was 23-years old, during a three-year stay in France at a Jesuit College, La Fléche, on the Loire.[6] In Book III of the *Treatise*, Hume declared that moral distinctions are not derived from unemotional reasoning; they are the result of what he called 'sympathy'—a capacity for sharing pleasure or pain. In a criticism of rationalist ethics, he explained, 'Our decisions concerning moral rectitude and depravity are evidently perceptions ... morality, therefore, is more properly felt than judg'd....' Hume's thesis has been aligned with aesthetics:[7] 'When reason has done all it can do to ascertain the facts, sentiment or taste must supervene to produce an idea of value, with nothing objective but the expression of a spectator's reaction to [hard] facts.' In this account of the roles of rationality and of feeling, in moral judgement, 'reason shows us *means*, sentiment selects *ends*.' Humean moral philosophy develops a complex account of sympathy: it is related not only to the motives of agents, but also to the world views of those persons affected by an action. And society is seen as supplying 'the additional force, ability and security' without which individual life cannot persist. These arguments are emphasised by Churchill, who concludes, 'If there is to be a social ethic of any force, it must be discovered as a necessary complement to an individual ethic.' 'Most persons would recognise,' he points out, '[it is] 'the inherent human affinity for relationships that is denied by social atomism, and the necessity for ethically interdependent relationships that is neglected by moral atomism.'

In light of these pleas for social ethics, how can we, for example, justify the heavy commitment to a philosophy of individualism as carried out in modern neonatal medicine? Jameton has recently[8] questioned the benevolence of the struggle in the US to keep individual marginally-viable neonates alive while ignoring the needs of families and community. The extravagant investment of resources in neonatal rescue, he points out, 'fosters an illusion that resources are not scarce.' The American neonatal intensive care unit (NICU) 'lives as if there were no budget, no global population and resource conflict, and no end of our ability to extend use of these means to save all infants victimized by poor public health, unfortunate genetics, and accidents of fate.' The truth is, he continues, 'by saving so few babies at such great expense while so many babies [throughout the world] die, the NICU represents an "island" mentality, suggesting that economic development improving the lives of a few people while neglecting a vast peripheral population is a sound strategy of coping with the global crisis of resources and population.' Jameton makes the gloomy prediction that the NICU will be 'a temporary historical phenomenon.'

'Looking ahead fifty years to a doubling of world population and even more greatly stressed total resources,' he finds it 'incredible to think that we will continue to invest social resources in such an extravagant and unbalanced way.' If we do, he foresees, 'we may well be charged by the next generations with inhumanity for our devotion.'

45

A 'win' in medical Russian roulette (1997)

Nothing exceeds like excess.

Anon

A large-scale randomised trial of extracorporeal membrane oxygenation (ECMO) for neonates with respiratory failure has been carried out in Britain, and early results were reported recently.[1] The long-awaited outcome of this study was published a full twenty years after the first successful adaptation of cardiopulmonary bypass for infants was described in the US in 1976.[2] During these two decades there were unrelenting arguments about whether or not there was enough evidence to justify wide use of the aggressive new technique.

The ECMO experience is a reminder that there are significant national differences in the factors and dynamics which come into play in the spread of high-cost, high-risk, high-tech modern interventions in medicine. The protracted period of controversy also calls attention to the kind of problems that turn up when the success of a new intervention depends on the skill of an individual doctor or on the smooth co-ordination of a highly-trained and experienced team of doctors, nurses, and technicians. The hard-won success of the experts at the end of a difficult learning period (their 'courage to fail') leads to a predicament that might be called 'technological entrapment:' Favourable local experience leads to intensely-held subjective convictions; any questions raised about the interpretation of results are taken as a personal affront. In the development of ECMO (and other 'desperation technologies [that] attract unusually positive assessment since they offer hope where there was no hope'[3]), it is easy to lose sight of an overriding question: How can we balance the technical challenge of perfecting hardware for life-support, as against medicine's humane imperative to avoid needless pain and suffering?

Following the introduction of the new technique in the US in the late 1970s, the survival rate of ECMO-treated infants improved dramatically, in association with increased practice in use of the procedure for desperately-ill full-term neonates. Activists argued that the effectiveness of ECMO was self-evident. A registry of ECMO-treated infants reported that 393 infants received this heroic treatment by the end of 1985; at the end of 1989 the number treated climbed to 3 577 patients—83% of infants reported to the registry survived.[4] But sceptics pointed to the difficulties of linking cause and magnitude of effect without concurrent controls at a time when overall neonatal survival rates were rising; and, more specifically, when survival with conventional ventilator treatment of respiratory failure was also increasing.[5-7]

The first randomised trial of ECMO was reported in 1984,[8] nine years after the procedure was introduced; five years later a second trial in the US was reported.[9] The favourable results in both of these exercises were questioned because too few patients were enrolled to provide reliable estimates of effect-size; and questions were also raised about the interpretation of the adaptive study-designs used (prior-outcome-dependent treatment allocation). A standard design was used in the third trial,[10] but, again, relatively few patients were enrolled, and the favourable results of that study were reported only in form of an abstract. Additionally, concerns were raised about numerous early and late adverse complications of the complex treatment, and about the inadequate number of concurrent conventionally-managed controls for follow-up.[11]

These cranky doubts about the ECMO programmes had little effect on slowing the spread of the technique in the US. On the contrary, there was external pressure to proceed forthwith. Four months before the results of the second randomised trial were published in a medical journal, the researchers were accused publicly of unethical conduct by denying 'life-saving therapy' (ECMO) to enrolled infants allocated to conventional management.[12]

In 1990, the Committee on Fetus and Newborn of the American Academy of Pediatrics acknowledged that 'new ECMO centers are evolving on the basis of current enthusiasm and without a thorough appreciation of the complexity, intensity, potential hazards, and uncertainties of this form of therapy.'[13] Curiously enough, the Committee recommended that the technique should be carried out only at major centres with 'active research programs,' and yet, nothing was said about the need for additional large-scale controlled trials. In the same year, the evidence then extant and the ethical issues involved in further clinical research of the topic were reviewed:[14] The authors listed a number of features in the ECMO experience that made it difficult, in their opinion, to evaluate the technique prospectively in controlled trials. They concluded that the experience with the development of this heroic treatment demonstrated the weaknesses of formal comparative trials as the ultimate basis for the resolution of medical disagreements. And they posited several values that would need to be sacrificed to attain greater certainty offered in randomised trials; among these is respect for the right of physicians to offer what they believe to be the best available treatment for their patients.

What was largely ignored in the debates about the use of ECMO in the US, was the role of market forces in the diffusion of this procedure which generated both profit and prestige at a time when competition between hospitals was heating up in that country. Ann Lennarson Greer, a sociologist, likened the hectic activity to an 'arms race'.[3] She pointed out that the need to transfer patients to another institution is often perceived as a threat by local doctors. '... [I]t is possible to imagine,' she noted, 'that neonatologists at a non-ECMO center might fear loss of referrals to a NICU [neonatal intensive care unit] having ECMO backup,' this leads to pressure for the establishment of local centres, each hoping to attract more patients. Moreover, the proliferation of the specialised centres in the US is not solely in the hands of doctors. 'Under market competition,' Greer noted, 'there is increased pressure [from managers] to direct funds to areas that enhance the hospital's visibility, market share, or potential to tap new markets.' Valerie Miké, a biostatistician, also questioned the quality of evidence used to justify the rapid diffusion of ECMO in the US.[15] She and her coworkers observed that the push for highly-visible development may also come from booster efforts of local government. For example, they came across a magazine advertisement in May 1990 paid for by the Board of City Development of an American city: 'Our ability to save struggling newborns with an ECMO Unit,' the ad boasted, 'makes [our city] one of the healthiest medical communities in the nation.'

Given the permissive views about rules of evidence in the development of desperation technologies and the operation of competitive market forces in the US, it is not surprising that ECMO has flourished in that country without further large-scale rigorous evaluation. Miké's group observed that 'of the more than 6 000 treated patients treated by mid-1992, only 40—less than 1%—were evaluated in a randomized trial.'

The spread of neonatal ECMO in Britain was, by contrast, very restrained. (In 1994–95, provision of ECMO centres was more than two and a half times more plentiful in the US as compared with the UK. In the US [1994], there were 75 ECMO centres[16] / 3 979 000 births[17] = ca 19 centres per 1 million births; compared with the UK's 5 centres [England, Scotland, and Wales] / 708 189 births, equivalent to 7 centres per 1 million births, A. Johnson, personal communication.) The UK Collaborative ECMO trial group explained[1] that the new technology was first used in Britain in 1989, but concerns about long-term disability, high costs, and uncertainty about effectiveness acted to slow acceptance. These fears led to an agreement to limit use only within a national randomised trial, and to define the primary outcome-of-interest as either death or severe disability (the latter to be assessed at the age of 1-year). Recruitment began on January 1, 1993 and was halted on November 23, 1995 when a decision was made that the trial provided a clear answer after the enrolment of 180 infants.

Although all survivors were not yet reviewed at age-1-year, the preliminary data suggested that rate of death or severe disability in the ECMO-treated group will be about one-half that in conventionally-managed babies (relative risk of outcome 0.54 [95% CI 0.36–0.80]). Since the preliminary rate of impairment among survivors was similar in the two groups (ECMO 11/43 [26%] *vs* conventional management 7/24 [29%]) it may turn out that the actual number of impaired survivors will be greater after ECMO treatment because of lowered mortality.

Roger Soll, an American neonatologist,[18] has praised the UK's ECMO centres for taking a more cautious approach than their US counterparts in adopting the controversial procedure. This is an encouraging sign, because it will be unfortunate if the British trial is condemned as an unethical effort to achieve little more than the 'greater certainty' denigrated in the US, six years earlier.[14] And it will be equally deplorable if the ECMO story is used to disparage a stern and time-honoured warning: Delay in mounting large-scale trials of a new treatment is a dangerous game. The medical profession would do well to remember that even in the admittedly hazardous game of Russian roulette with a six-shooter, in a long series of plays, 5-out-of-6 spins of the gun's cylinder are expected to end in a 'win' for a gullible player—but when the 1-in-6 loss occurs, it is devastating.

Have we already forgotten the lesson taught by the hapless use of DES (diethylstilbestrol) over a period of 20 years, to improve pregnancy outcome?[19] That unhappy episode demonstrated just how catastrophic a loss can be when 'greater certainty' is eschewed out of respect for the prerogative of physicians to offer what they *believe* to be the best available treatment.

If there are doubts that such mishaps (the medical analogues of 'friendly fire' disasters in conventional warfare) can and do still occur, the uncritical optimism was dispelled by some recent gloomy news. The safety of pulmonary artery (PA) catheterisation for monitoring haemodynamic events in seriously-ill patients has been questioned. (More than 1-million PA catheters have been sold each year in the US, since the specially-designed balloon-tipped devices were introduced in 1970.) The technique, it turns out, was never subjected to rigorous tests. For example, an RCT, attempted in 1991, was terminated because most doctors were so convinced the procedure was safe they refused to allow their patients to be randomised. Now, after 26 years of an enormous world-wide experience, a large prospective observational cohort study (of 5 735 critically ill patients receiving care in an intensive care unit in five US teaching hospitals between 1989 and 1994) has found a measurable increase in mortality associated with PA catheterisation.[21] And there is now a clamour for a proper randomised trial of the procedure.[22]

The more things change, sadly, the more they are the same.

Reply by John D. Lantos:

(1997)

Disabuse: To present your neighbour with another and better error than one which he has deemed it advantageous to embrace.

Ambrose Bierce's *Devil's Dictionary*

Silverman sets about to disabuse readers of misperceptions they may have gained from reading an essay that Joel Frader and I wrote in 1990.[1] In particular, Silverman worries that we might condemn as unethical efforts to achieve greater certainty than was available through careful analysis of retrospective studies and small prospective studies. He is also concerned that we did not adequately consider the role of market forces in the diffusion of ECMO in the United States.

By 1993, when the UK Collaborative ECMO trial was initiated, it had been seventeen years since the first successful use of ECMO in neonates.[2] Analysis of three small randomised trials had concluded that ECMO was superior to maximal ventilatory support for infants with meconium aspiration and persistent pulmonary hypertension, congenital diaphragmatic hernia or pneumonia and sepsis when those infants met rigorous criteria for severe respiratory failure. More than 7 500 babies had been treated with ECMO in 75 programmes in the United States and 17 programmes in other countries.[3] Nevertheless, physicians in the UK were uncertain whether the data on the efficacy of ECMO were convincing, and set about to do another randomised clinical trial.

Whenever we consider a randomised trial, we must ask whether we are in a state of genuine uncertainty about the relative merits of the two arms of the trial. If we are not, then it is unethical to randomise patients. Instead, we have an obligation to offer the therapy which is more beneficial. If we are genuinely uncertain, than a randomised trial is not only permissible but may be obligatory as a way of maximising the chances that our patients get the best available treatment. Randomisation, though always problematic, may thus sometimes be the best approach for both the treatment of patients and the evaluation of an innovative therapy. But not always.

Whenever anybody wants to make an argument for greater use of randomised controlled trials, they cite the diethylstilbestrol (DES) debacle. This is a bit misleading. A randomised controlled trial of DES done at the University of Chicago showed that DES was ineffective in preventing premature labour,[4] and this was part of the reason why the use of DES declined. The trial did not include vaginal adenocarcinoma in the offspring of treated women as an endpoint. Most trials do not examine outcomes in the offspring of treated patients. The association between DES and vaginal adenocarcinoma was discovered using a retrospective case control study design.[5] Even randomised trials have limitations. We live in a world where knowledge is always imperfect, where innovation is always associated with peril. One of those perils is the overuse of randomised trials.

In his book on the evaluation of thrombolytic therapies, Brody[6] gives a striking example of the unethical use of randomised trials. Long after intracoronary streptokinase had been shown to be efficacious in reducing mortality from acute myocardial infarction, studies continued to be done that randomised patients to a new intervention or a placebo. Brody argues that such trials for thrombolytic therapy led to the avoidable and unnecessary deaths of 497 people. These 497 people were those who were given placebos in trials of intravenous thrombolytics after intra-coronary streptokinase had been proven effective and had been approved by the FDA. Brody suggests that, since proven treatment was available, placebo controlled trials were unethical. Each of these studies was subsequently published in peer-reviewed journals without apparent concern about the ethics of study design. We seem to have become so enamoured of randomised trials that we can no longer see some of the problems and conflicts that they raise.

More certainty is always better than less certainty but at some point, we need to decide that we are certain enough. The UK ECMO trial makes us more certain that ECMO works, but are we certain enough? One way to think about this would be to ask whether another study to confirm the results of the UK Collaborative ECMO trial would be ethical at this point. After all, the scientific method would seem to demand that experiments be repeated to make certain that the results are valid. By this argument, we should do another study. But most doctors, I imagine, would be reluctant to participate in another trial. While not completely certain, they are certain enough. In the United States, most doctors were certain enough before the UK trial.

There will always be tensions in the development of new technologies. Market forces in the United States created an environment in which profits could be made by successfully marketing hospitals and health care systems. In a culture enamoured of high technology and the appearance of progress, successful marketing often demanded that hospitals tout the 'latest' medical developments, even if they were not the best medical developments. But market forces are not always evil. In Britain, by contrast, the lack of market forces and the administrative structures for the evaluation of new therapies may delay the introduction of beneficial therapies. Market forces sometimes demand that unnecessary trials be conducted. Brody demonstrates that a number of unnecessary or unethical trials of thrombolytic therapies were conducted in both the United States and Europe primarily because different drug companies wanted to prove that their product was efficacious.

In 1990, Frader and I[1] argued that randomised controlled trials involved a number of trade-offs, and that, although they are epistemologically pleasing in a way that other study designs are not, they may not always be necessary, desirable, or practical to conduct. At one level, our argument was simply a practical one. We can never evaluate every innovation using randomised controlled trials because, if we tried, we would always be doing trials. Innovation is a constant and intrinsic aspect of modern medicine. Most innovations are minor variations on a theme, but even they change the mix of available therapies.

At some point, we have to make a judgement about whether or not enough is known about a treatment to deem it better, worse, or about the same as another treatment. When is a therapy ever evaluated enough? When can we say, for sure, that the definitive study has been done and that further study will add no new knowledge? The answer, clearly, is never. There are always innovations, new indications, new drugs or devices that can be given in new combinations. In an epistemologically perfect world, each combination of interventions should be rigorously evaluated against each other possible combination of interventions. Every new drug or device would change the mix, so that, with each advance, testing would need to start anew. Only then would we know, without dogma or bias, what was or was not effective.

We would also be paralysed. Innovation would stop. The evaluation of innovation would become the enemy of innovation.

A deeply-held dogma is a terrible thing We would all prefer to be open-minded than to be dogmatic, to consider the evidence fairly, to be rational rather than biased. And yet, it is often difficult to disentangle dogma from conviction, belief from bias, and faith from knowledge.

Silverman's editorial about ECMO states that early in the days of ECMO, 'activists' argued that the effectiveness of ECMO was 'self-evident.' That oversimplifies the story a bit. ECMO investigators were rigorous in their evaluation of ECMO and their publication of results. They published their eligibility criteria, their outcomes, and their complications. They refined their indications and their techniques based on collected experience, and they conducted two randomised controlled trials. Their only sin was that they became convinced of the benefits of ECMO before some statisticians were convinced, and so, felt that it would be unethical to continue to randomise patients to an inferior therapy. The question is not whether ECMO has been evaluated but whether it had been evaluated enough.

The design of the British trial drew heavily on this accumulated experience. Techniques, eligibility criteria, and contraindications were all based on the previous world-wide experience. And the results were, predictably, the same as the results of other countries and other centres. In the UK Collaborative ECMO trial, 32% of babies in the ECMO arm died, compared with 59% of babies in the conventional arm. There were 24 'excess' deaths in the conventional arm.[7] I'm not sure how I would feel if I was one of the parents whose baby received conventional therapy and died. Of more concern, it is not clear, from the study report, what happened to babies whose parents did not want their babies to be in the study. Presumably, they received 'conventional' therapy, and presumably, the only way they could have gained access to ECMO would have been to agree to be randomised.

I would have suggested the opposite, that all the evidence to date suggested that ECMO was more effective than 'conventional' therapy and so, ECMO should have been the default treatment of choice. As the trial was designed, there was an implicit element of coercion in this study design.

I think that the data that were available in the early 1990s on the benefits for ECMO were convincing. I have concern about informed consent and possible coercion in the UK study. For these reasons, if I was on an ethics review panel, I would not have approved the trial.

Citations

The 'Fumes....' essays were published originally without titles in the 'From our correspondents' section of *Paediatric and Perinatal Epidemiology*, as noted in parentheses immediately under each of the numbered titles below. Superscripts in the text refer to the numbers listed here under each essay. See alphabetised Bibliography for complete references.

Introduction

(Adapted from the 1994 Windermere Lecture at the 66th annual meeting of the British Paediatric Association; published in *Archives of Disease in Childhood* 1994; **71**: 261–265)

1. Callahan, 1990.
2. Silverman, 1980.
3. Rothman, 1978.
4. Postman, 1992.
5. Doxiadis, 1987.
6. Lehrer, 1965.
7. von Clausewitz, 1952.
8. Freidson, 1972.
9. Dworkin, 1993.
10. Engelhardt, 1982.
11. Brody, 1992.

1 Selective ethics

(*Paediatric and Perinatal Epidemiology* 1987; **1**: 10–12)

1. Smithells, 1975.
2. Nicholson, 1986.
3. Wilder, 1942.

(1997)

1. Cryotherapy for Retinopathy..., 1996.
2. Palmer, 1996.

2   Does a difference make a difference?

(*Paediatric and Perinatal Epidemiology* 1987; **1**: 137–138)

1. Tukey, 1962.
2. Shaw GB, 1911.
3. Gardner and Altman, 1986.
4. Mainland, 1984.
5. Schneiderman MA, 1964.
6. Comroe, 1977.
7. Torrance *et al.*, 1972.
8. Burroughs, 1900.

(1997)

1. Guyatt *et al.*, 1995.
2. Cook RJ. and Sackett, 1995.

3   Prescription for disaster

(*Paediatric and Perinatal Epidemiology* 1988; **2**: 5–7)

1. Bates, 1980.
2. Stinson and Stinson, 1983.
3. Lyon, 1985.
4. Gustaitis and Young, 1986
5. Guillemin and Holmstrom, 1986.
6. Frohock, 1986
7. Henaean, 1979.
8. Kulkarni *et al.*, 1978.
9. Sameroff and Chandler, 1975.
10. Marris, 1974.

(1997)

1. Stinson and Stinson, 1983.
2. Alecson, 1995.
3. Horbar and Chandler, 1997.

4   Therapeutic mystique

(*Paediatric and Perinatal Epidemiology* 1988; **2**: 116–118)

1. Volgyesi, 1954.
2. Haygarth, 1800.
3. Shapiro, 1960.
4. Leader, 1970.
5. Gribben, 1981.

6. Asher, 1972.
7. Wolf S, 1962.
8. Freedman, 1987.
9. Shaw LW and Chalmers, 1970.
10. Marquis, 1983.
11. Balint, 1957.
12. Houston, 1938.
13. Fried, 1974.
14. Parsons, 1951.
15. Bracken, 1987.
16. Blum *et al.*, 1987.

(1997)

1. Johansson *et al.*, 1997.
2. Kolata, February 12, 1997.

5   Humane limits

(*Paediatric and Perinatal Epidemiology* 1988; **2**: 208–210)

1. Konner, 1987
2. Thomas, 1987.
3. Sternberg, 1924.
4. Treuherz, 1987.
5. Lyon, 1985.
6. Bloom, 1986.
7. Singer , 1987.
8. Murton *et al.*, 1987.
9. Thoreau, 1966.

(1997)

1. Tin *et al.*, 1997.
2. Fetus and Newborn Committee of the American Academy of Pediatrics, 1994
3. Fetus and Newborn Committee of the American Academy of Pediatrics, 1995.
4. Paneth *et al.*, (in preparation).
5. Ellul, 1980.

6   Intruding in private tragedies

(*Paediatric and Perinatal Epidemiology* 1988; **2**: 308–310)

1. Scott, 1987.
2. Comment, 1981.

3. Ferriman, 1981.
4. Excerpts, 1981.
5. Levine C *et al.*, 1984.
6. Infant Bioethics Task Force, 1984.
7. Churchill, 1980.
8. Galbraith, 1977.
9. Guillemin, 1984.
10. Mother (A), 1984.

(1997)

1. Clark, 1996.
2. Harrison, 1996.
3. Moskowitz and Nelson, 1995.
4. Becker *et al.*, 1993.

7 The glut of information

(*Paediatric and Perinatal Epidemiology* 1989; **3**: 4–5)

1. Healy, 1976.
2. Durack, 1978.
3. de S Price, 1981.
4. Anonymous, 1975.
5. Burman, 1982.
6. Goldsmith, 1759.
7. Policy Research Incorporated, 1979.
8. Paterson and Bailar, 1985.
9. Rennie, 1986.
10. Lock, 1985.
11. Bailar and Paterson 1985.
12. Sackett *et al.*, 1985a.
13. Virgo, 1977.
14. Bruer, 1982.
15. Bailar, 1982.
16. First (The) International Congress on Peer Review, 1989.
17. Peters and Ceci, 1982.
18. Armstrong, 1984.
19. Walster and Cleary, 1970.

(1997)

1. Rennie and Flanagin, 1994.
2. Judson, 1994.
3. Smith and Rennie, 1995.
4. Roszak, 1991.
5. Shenk, 1997.

8 Betting on specified horses

(*Paediatric and Perinatal Epidemiology* 1989; **3**: 109–110)

1. Medawar, 1984.
2. Medawar, 1969.
3. Galton, 1872.
4. Tukey, 1977.
5. Meittinen, 1985.
6. Louis *et al.*, 1984.

(1997)

1. Wilford, 1995.
2. Zupancic *et al.*, 1997.
3. Levenson, 1994.
10. Kolata, 1995.

9 Begin with 'If....'

(*Paediatric and Perinatal Epidemiology* 1989; **3**: 242–245)

1. Freirich and Gehan, 1979.
2. Kuban *et al.*, 1988.
3. Hill, 1962.
4. Sackett, 1979.
5. Edlund *et al.*, 1985.
6. Sackett *et al.*, 1985b.
7. Dudley, 1987.
8. Mainland, 1984.
9. Bailar, 1985.
10. Mainland, 1960.
11. FDA, 1977.
12. Jennett, 1987.

(1997)

1. Moore DS, 1979.
2. Ellenberg, 1994.
3. Dudley, 1987.

10 Archie's scepticism

(*Paediatric and Perinatal Epidemiology* 1989; **3**: 357–359)

1. Cochrane, 1972.
2. Mather *et al.*, 1971.
3. Marquis, 1983.

4. Gifford, 1986.
5. Vere, 1983.

(1997)

1. Alvarez-Dardet and Ruiz, 1993.
2. Cochrane, 1979.
3. Chalmers I *et al.*, 1989.
4. Editorial, 1992.
5. Chalmers I *et al.*, 1992.
6. Maynard and Chalmers, 1997.

11 Arbitrary vs discretionary decisions

(*Paediatric and Perinatal Epidemiology* 1990; **4**: 4–6)

1. Cook DJ *et al.*, 1995.
2. Beauchamp and Childress, 1979.
3. Shorter, 1975.
4. Budin, 1907.
5. Cone, 1985.
6. Boyle *et al.*, 1983.
7. Buchanan, 1987.
8. Report, 1988.

(1997)

1. Williams, 1997.

12 Bioengineering

(*Paediatric and Perinatal Epidemiology* 1990; **4**: 129–131)

1. Tredgold, 1987.
2. Rabi, 1975.
3. Bacon, 1878.
4. Descartes, 1956.
5. Cohen IB, 1985.
6. Sass, 1988.
7. Singer and Wells, 1984.
8. Pauly, 1987.
9. Healy MJR, 1978.

(1997)

1. Kolata, February 23, 1997.
2. Kimbrell, 1993.
3. Jonas, 1984.

13 '....disavowing the tree'

(*Paediatric and Perinatal Epidemiology* 1990; **4**: 255–258)

1. Fletcher, 1907.
2. Vollrath, 1989.
3. Leary, 1989.
4. Marquis, 1983.
5. Cahn, 1972.
6. Chalmers, I and Silverman, 1987.

(1997)

1. Silverman, 1997.
2. Sigerist, 1941.
3. Jonas, 1969.

14 Diffusing responsibility

(*Paediatric and Perinatal Epidemiology* 1990; **4**: 402–406)

1. Hayek, 1960.
2. Manchester, 1988.
3. Annotation, 1982.
4. Hershey and Fisher, 1982.
5. Apgar, 1953.
6. Campbell, 1988.
7. Annotation, 1988.
8. Walker, 1988.
9. Sass, 1988.
10. Dyson, 1984

Weil's reply

1. Koshland, 1988.

15 Hawthorne effects

(*Paediatric and Perinatal Epidemiology* 1991; **5**: 4–7)

1. Edlund *et al.*, 1985.
2. Snow, 1927.
3. Roethlisberger and Dickson, 1939.
4. Whyte, 1961.
5. Last, 1983.
6. Rosenthal and Jacobson, 1968.
7. Parsons, 1951.
8. Cassileth *et al.*, 1982.

9. Findley, 1953.
10. Epstein and Pinski, 1961.

(1997)

1. Nickel, 1997.
2. Cobb *et al.*, 1959.

16 Power plays

(*Paediatric and Perinatal Epidemiology* 1991; **5**: 133–136)

1. Lewis, 1952.
2. Pless, 1983.
3. Doe (*in re*), 1982.
4. Department of Health and Human Services, 1984.
5. Holder, 1983
6. American Academy of Pediatrics v heckler, 1983.
7. US Child Abuse, 1984.
8. Gerry and Nimz, 1987.
9. Cohen CB *et al.*, 1987.
10. Kopelman *et al.*, 1988.

(1997)

1. Murray, 1994.
2. Nelson, 1992.
3. Harrison, 1993.

17 Unbridled enthusiasm

(*Paediatric and Perinatal Enthusiasm* 1991; **5**: 258–260)

1. Insight Team, 1979
2. Kelsey, 1963.
3. Editorial, 1989.
4. Kolata, 1989.
5. Braff, 1989.
6. Boston Interhospital Virus Study Group, 1975.
7. Moses, 1984.
8. Grace *et al.*, 1966.
9. Chalmers, TC *et al.*, 1972.
10. Bearman *et al.*, 1974.

(1997)

1. Eisenberg *et al.*, 1993.

2. Campion, 1993.
3. Holmes, 1996.

18 Caring and curing

(*Paediatric and Perinatal Epidemiology* 1991; **5**: 373–376)

1. Webster, 1995.
2. Dubos, 1979.
3. Scheiber and Poulier, 1988.
4. Callahan, 1990.
5. Skrabanek and McCormick, 1989.
6. Nader, 1975.
7. US Congressional Office of Technology Assessment, 1988.
8. Eisenberg L, 1990.

(1997)

1. Lamm, 1994.

19 On the edge

(*Paediatric and Perinatal Epidemiology* 1992; **6**: 14–17)

1. Hull, 1988.
2. Cone, 1985.
3. Ballantyne, 1902.
4. Crosse, 1945.
5. Chapin, 1900.
6. Blair VP, 1904.
7. Stahlman, 1989.

(1997)

1. Quinn, 1994.
2. Rawls, 1993.
3. Renzong, 1987.

20 Informing and consenting

(*Paediatric and Perinatal Epidemiology* 1992; **6**: 316–321)

1. Faden and Beauchamp, 1986.
2. Katz, 1972.
3. Beecher, 1966.
4. Stewart, 1966.
5. Streptomycin in Tuberculosis Trial Committee, 1948.

6. Hill, 1990.
7. Simes *et al.*, 1986.
8. Edlund *et al.*, 1985.
9. Harth amd Thong, 1990.

Weil's reply

1. Miller, 1981.
2. Lomas, 1989.
3. Bartholome, 1989.

(1997)

1. Silverman, 1995.
2. Segelov *et al.*, 1992.

21 Lifesavers

(*Paediatric and Perinatal Epidemiology* 1992; **6**: 398–401)

1. Nuland, 1994.
2. Gustaitis and Young, 1986.
3. Frohock, 1986.
4. Shepard, 1990.
5. Guillemin and Holmstrom, 1986.
6. Candee *et al.*, 1982.
7. Kohlberg, 1976.
8. Rest, 1979.
9. Emery, 1990.

(1997)

1. Nuland, 1994.
2. Skolnick, 1996.

22 Belief and disbelief

(*Paediatric and Perinatal Epidemiology* 1993; **7**: 5–7)

1. Mortimer, 1994.
2. Freidson, 1972.
3. Hughes, 1958.
4. Larson, 1978.
5. Parsons, 1951.
6. Deber and Thompson, 1990.

(1997)

1. Greer, 1994.

23 Preferences

(Paediatric and Perinatal Epidemiology 1993; **7**: 152–155)

1. Boston Women's Health Book Collective, 1971.
2. Eddy, 1990.
3. Wennberg, 1990.
4. Wennberg *et al.*, 1988.
5. Brewin and Bradley, 1989.
6. Janis and Mann, 1977.
7. Korn and Baumrind, 1991.

(1997)

1. Till *et al.*, 1992.
2. Henshaw *et al.*, 1993.
3. Silverman, 1996.
4. Paulos, 1992.

24 Bradford Hill's doubts

(Paediatric and Perinatal Epidemiology 1993; **7**: 230–232)

1. Hill, 1962.
2. Hill, 1937.
3. Medical Research Council, 1948.
4. Hill, 1990.

(1997)

1. Meisel and Roth, 1981.
2. Counsell and Sandercock, 1997.
3. Armitage, 1992.

25 More informative abstracts

(Paediatric and Perinatal Epidemiology 1993; **7**: 349–351)

1. Pauli, 1990.
2. Durack, 1978.
3. Price de S, 1963.
4. Warren, 1981.
5. Bernier and Yerkey, 1979.
6. Sackett *et al.*, 1985b.
7. Ertl, 1969.
8. Huth, 1987.
9. *Ad hoc* Working Group, 1987.

10 Mulrow....., 1988.
11. Haynes *et al.*, 1990.

(1997)

1. [The] Standards of Reporting Trials Group, 1994.
2. Society for Pediatric Epidemiologic Research, 1991.
3. Gøtzsche, 1989.
4. Schulz *et al.*, 1995.
5. Working Group, 1994.
6. Begg *et al.*, 1996
7. Altman DG, 1996.

26 Pain control in neonates

(*Paediatric and Perinatal Epidemiology* 1994; **8**: 22–25)

1. Shipley, 1979.
2. Anand *et al.*, 1987a.
3. Pernick, 1985.
4. Lawson, 1986.
5. Anand *et al.*, 1987b.
6. Forfar and Campbell, 1987.
7. Wilkinson, 1987.
8. *Daily Mail*, 1987.
9. All Party Parliamentary Pro-Life Group, 1987.
10. Editorial, 1987.
11. Walton, 1987.
12. Braine, 1988.
13. Anand *et al.*, 1990.
14. Anand and Hickey, 1992.
15. Quinn *et al.*, 1993.

(1997)

1. Wolf, 1993.
2. Partridge and Wall, 1997.
3. Taddio *et al.*, 1997.
4. Schechter *et al.*, 1997.

27 Miraculous cures

(*Paediatric and Perinatal Epidemiology* 1994; **8**: 140–143)

1. Socrates, 1991.
2. Wachter de, 1992.

3. Navarro, 1992.
4. Shorter, 1992.
5. Hilgard, 1980.
6. Darnton, 1968.
7. Gould, 1991.
8. Popper, 1962.

(1997)

1. Miller, 1995.

28 Observer bias

(*Paediatric and Perinatal Epidemiology* 1994; **8**: 258–261)

1. Wallace, 1965.
2. Hardwick...., 1964.
3. Schilpp, 1974.
4. Popper, 1962.
5. Kuhn, 1970.
6. Asher, 1958–59.
7. Ederer, 1975.
8. Rennie, 1991.
9. Cantekin *et al.*, 1991.

(1997)

1. Greenberg and Fisher, 1994.

29 The gatekeeper's brouhaha

(*Paediatric and Perinatal Epidemiology* 1994; **8**: 359–362)

1. Rennie, 1991.
2. Report by the Committee on Government Operations, 1989.
3. Bell, 1992.
4. Mandel *et al.*, 1987.
5. Cantekin *et al.*, 1990
6. Office of Scientific Integrity Inquiry, 1990.
7. Cantekin *et al.*, 1991.
8. Etzel *et al.*, 1992.

(1997)

1. Hall, 1997.
2. Dreyfuss, 1997.

30 Creatures of bounded rationality

(*Paediatric and Perinatal Epidemiology* 1995; **9**: 30–32)

1. Proust, 1932.
2. Janis and Mann, 1977.
3. Tversky and Kahneman,1981.
4. Georgescu-Roegen, 1974.
5. Escobar *et al.*, 1991.
6. Simon, 1976.

(1997)

1. Feinstein, 1992.
2. Fahey *et al.*, 1995.
3. Milne and Sackett, 1995.

31 Champing at the bit

(*Paediatric and Perinatal Epidemiology* 1995; **9**: 130–138)

1. Silverman *et al.*, 1956.
2. Miké, 1989.
3. Aboulker and Swart, 1993.
4. Altman LK, 1993.

(1997)

1. Singer, 1993.

32 Piecemeal skirmishes

(*Paediatric and Perinatal Epidemiology* 1995; **9**: 250–253)

1. Terry, 1942.
2. Watts, 1992.
3. Kinsey, 1955.
4. Cryotherapy for Retinopathy of Prematurity Cooperative Group, 1988.
5. Owens and Owens, 1949.
6. Institute of Medicine, 1986.
7. Saugstad, 1992.
8. Sullivan and Newton, 1988.
9. Sullivan, 1992.
10. Lakatos *et al.*, 1986.
11. Shenai *et al.*, 1987.
12. Hallman *et al.*, 1992.
13. Palmer *et al.*, 1991.

14. Cryotherapy for Retinopathy of Prematurity Cooperative Group, 1993.
15. Hack and Fanaroff, 1993.
16. Pocock, 1983.

(1997)

1. Saunders *et al.*, 1997.
2. Lockeand Reese, 1952.
3. Seiberth *et al.*, 1994.
4. Gilbert *et al.*, 1997.

33 Resolution of insoluble dilemmas

(*Paediatric and Perinatal Epidemiology* 1995; **9**: 370–379)

1. Bascom, 1975.
2. Editorial, 1988.
3. Hack and Fanaroff, 1993.
4. Walker, 1988.
5. Frohock, 1986.
6. Lilienfeld and Pasamanick, 1955.
7. Blair E and Stanley, 1988.
8. Ounsted, 1987.
9. Ounsted *et al.*, 1984.
10. Sameroff and Chandler, 1975.
11. Werner *et al.*, 1971.
12. Thucydides, 1993.

Sinclair and Fowlie's reply:

1. Adebayu, personal communication.
2. Duc and Sinclair, 1992a.
3. Duc and Sinclair, 1992b.
4. Saigal *et al.*, 1996.
5. Saigal *et al.*, 1995a.

Watts and Saigal's reply:

1. King, 1992.
2. Rhoden, 1986.
3. Brody, 1989.
4. Botkin, 1990.
5. Fetus and Newborn Committee, 1994.
6. Lilienfeld and Pasamanick, 1955.
7. Ounsted *et al.*, 1984.
8. Robertson *et al.*, 1992.
9. Pinto-Martin *et al.*, 1995.

10. Saigal *et al.*, 1995b.
11. Saigal *et al.*, 1996.

34 'Fixing' human reproduction

(*Paediatric and Perinatal Epidemiology* 1996; **10**: 17–20)

1. Ludmerer, 1972.
2. Darwin and Wallace, 1858.
3. Wolpert, 1993.
4. Hofstadter, 1955.
5. *Buck v Bell*, 1927.
6. Seller, 1993.
7. Zenzes...., 1992.

(1997)

1. Pernick, 1996.

35 Justice defined as fairness

(*Paediatric and Perinatal Epidemiology* 1996; **10**: 124–127)

1. Worster, 1992.
2. Budin, 1907.
3. Hack and Fanaroff, 1989.
4. Allen *et al.*, 1993.
5. Hack and Fanaroff, 1993.
6. Fetus and Newborn Committee, 1993.
7. Lynn and De Grazia, 1991.
8. Lidz and Meisel, 1983.
9. Rawls, 1993.
10. Dworkin, 1994.
11. Dworkin, 1993.

(1997)

1. Institute of Medicine..., 1997.
2. Editorial, 1997.
3. McCarthy, 1997.
4. Harrison, 1993.

36 'Methods-based' reviews

(*Paediatric and Perinatal Epidemiology* 1996; **10**: 264–267)

1. Percival, 1803.
2. Faden and Beauchamp, 1986.

3. Levine RJ, 1981.
4. Trials of War Criminals, 1949.
5. Ladimer, 1963.
6. World Medical Association, 1964.
7. World Medical Association, 1975.
8. Frankel, 1975.
9. McNeill, 1993.
10. Annas, 1988.
11. Kavanaugh *et al.*, 1979.
12. Alberti, 1995.
13. Foster, 1995.
14. Rutstein, 1969.
15. Altman DG, 1994.
16. Prescott, 1977.

(1997)

1. World Medical Association....., 1997.
2. Amdur and Biddle, 1997.
3. Weiss, 1989.
4. Porter, 1997.

37 Non-replication of the replicable

(*Paediatric and Perinatal Epidemiology* 1996; **10**: 406–409)

1. Konner, 1982.
2. Haines and Jones, 1994.
3. Drummond and Wilbraham, 1940.
4. Cohen MM....., 1960.
5. Ambrus *et al.*, 1963.
6. Ambrus *et al.*, 1966.
7. Ambrus *et al.*, 1977.
8. Leroux *et al.*, 1976.
9. Dancis, 1968.
10. Lakatos *et al.*, 1982.
11. Watts, 1992.
12. Lakatos and Oroszlan, 1994.
13. Guyatt, 1991.

(1997)

1. Fisher, 1926.
2. Fisher, 1960.
3. Mainland, 1960.
4. Dworkin, 1991.

38 Who defines 'futility' ?

(*Paediatric and Perinatal Epidemiology* 1997; **11**: 21–24)

1. Ramsey, 1970.
2. Hey, 1980.
3. Paris *et al.*, 1990.
4. Editorial Board, 1990.
5. Fleischman, 1993.
6. Phoon, 1993.
7. King, 1992.
8. Tocqueville, 1988.
9. Fox and Swazey, 1992a.
10. Annas, 1994.
11. Annas..., 1996.

Goldworth and Benitz's reply:

(*Paediatric and Perinatal Epidemiology* 1997; **11**: 377–378)

1. Paris *et al.*, 1990.
2. Goldworth and Benitz, 1995.
3. Fleischman, 1990.

39 Fitting targets to holes

(*Paediatric and Perinatal Epidemiology* 1997; **11**: 136–138)

1. Boorstin, 1994.
2. Castiglioni, 1941.
3. Berendes, 1966.
4. Hutchison, 1966.
5. Peto *et al.*, 1993.
6. Jolley, 1993.

(1997)

1. MacDonald, 1996
2. Blair and Stanley, 1988.
3. Perlman, 1997.

40 Medical 'manners' on trial

(*Paediatric and Perinatal Epidemiology* 1997; **11**: 380–384)

1. Moulton, 1924.
2. Kidder, 1995.
3. Bray, 1995.

4. Callahan, 1994.
5. Katz, 1972.
6. Fox and Swazey, 1992b.

(1997)

1. Bray, 1997.

41 Sanction of whose beliefs and values?

(*Paediatric and Perinatal Epidemiology* 1998; **12**: 2–4)

1. Mumford, 1951.
2. Applebaum *et al.*, 1987.
3. Katz, 1984.
4. Veatch, 1995.
5. Schneiderman LJ *et al.*, 1993.
6. Engelhardt, 1982.

(1997)

1. Cook DJ *et al.*, 1995.
2. Moscowitz and Nelson, 1995.
3. SUPPORT (The)...., 1995.
4. Annas, 1996.

42 Mindless existence

(*Paediatric and Perinatal Epidemiology*, in press)

1. Callahan, 1993.
2. Associated Press, 1995.
3. Wachter de, 1992.
4. Simons, 1995.
5. Final report, 1987.
6. Maas van der, 1995.
7. Blendon *et al.*, 1992.
8. Claiborne, 1992.
9. Singer, 1994.
10. *Airedale NH Trust v. Bland*, 1993.
11. Stevenson *et al.*, 1986.
12. Dworkin, 1993.

(1997)

1. Hendin, 1997.
2. Lynn, 1997.

3. Heide van der *et al.*, 1997
4. Churchill and King, 1997.

43 Interventions on an unprecedented scale

(*Paediatric and Perinatal Epidemiology*, in press)

1. Lasagna, 1964.
2. Jonas, 1984.
3. Thomas, 1983.
4. Moore, 1995.
5. Cardiac Arrhythmia Suppression Trial, 1989.
6. Cardiac Arrhythmia Suppression Trial, 1992.
7. Jonas, 1969.

44 Preoccupation with 'autonomy'

(*Paediatric and Perinatal Epidemiology*, in press)

1. Hume, 1978.
2. Etzioni, 1987.
3. Nelson, 1992.
4. Churchill, 1994.
5. Murray, 1994.
6. MacIntyre, 1965.
7. Raphael, 1973.
8. Jameton, 1995.

45 A 'win' in medical Russian roulette

(*Paediatric and Perinatal Epidemiology* 1997; **11**: 260–268)

1. UK Collaborative ECMO Trial Group, 1996.
2. Bartlett *et al.*, 1976.
3. Greer, 1993.
4. Neonatal Extracorporeal Life Support Registry, 1990.
5. Davis *et al.*, 1988.
6. Ortega *et al.*, 1988.
7. Dworetz *et al.*, 1989.
8. Bartlett *et al.*, 1985.
9. O'Rourke *et al.*, 1989.
10. Bifano *et al.*, 1992.
11. Elliott, 1991.
12. Knox, 1989.
13. Fetus and Newborn Committee, 1990.

14. Lantos and Frader, 1990.
15. Miké *et al.*, 1993.
16. Kanto, 1994
17. Guyer *et al.*, 1994.
18. Johnson, 1996.
19. Soll, 1996.
20. Goldstein *et al.*, 1989.
21. Connors *et al.*, 1996.
22. Sandham *et al.*, 1996.

Lantos' reply:

1. Lantos and Frader, 1990.
2. Bartlett *et al.*, 1976.
3. Kanto, 1994.
4. Dieckman *et al.*, 1953.
5. Herbst *et al.*, 1971.
6. Brody, 1996.
7. UK Collaborative ECMO Trial Group, 1996.

Bibliography

Aboulker JP, Swart AM. Preliminary analysis of the Concorde trial (letter). *Lancet* 1993; **341**: 889–890.

Adebayu Ayede, personal communication.

Ad Hoc Working Group for Critical Appraisal of the Medical Literature. A proposal for more informative abstracts of clinical articles. *Annals of Internal Medicine* 1987; **106**: 598–604.

Airedale N.H.Trust v. Bland 1993, Weekly Law Reports, pp. 316–400.

Alberti KGMM. Local research committees. Time to grab several bulls by the horns. *British Medical Journal* 1995; **311**: 639–640.

Alecson DG. Lost Lullaby. Berkeley: University of California Press, 1995.

Allen MC, Donohue PK, Dusman AE. The limit of viability—neonatal outcome of infants born at 22 to 25 weeks gestation. *New England Journal of Medicine* 1993; **329**: 1597–1601.

All Party Parliamentary Pro-Life Group. Press release for immediate publication. July 29,1987.

Altman DG. The scandal of poor medical research. *British Medical Journal* 1994; **308**: 283–284.

Altman DG. Better reporting of randomised controlled trials: the CONSORT statement. *British Medical Association* 1996; **313**: 570–571.

Altman LK. AIDS study casts doubt on value of hastened drug approval in U.S. *New York Times* April 6, 1993.

Alvarez-Dardet C, Ruiz MT. Thomas McKeown and Archibald Cochrane: a journey through the diffusion of their ideas. *British Medical Journal* 1993; **306**: 1252–1254.

Ambrus CM, Weintraub DH, Dunphy D *et al.* Studies on hyaline membrane disease. I. The fibrinolysin system in pathogenesis and therapy. *Pediatrics* 1963; **32**: 10–24.

Ambrus CM, Weintraub DH, Ambrus JL. Studies on hyaline membrane disease. III. Therapeutic trial of urokinase-activated human plasmin. *Pediatrics* 1966; **38**: 231–243.

Ambrus CM, Choi TS, Cunnanan E *et al.* Prevention of hyaline membrane disease with plasminogen. A cooperative study. *Journal of the American Medical Association* 1977; **237**: 1837–1841.

Amdur RJ, Biddle C. Institutional review board approval and publication of human research results. *Journal of the American Medical Association* 1997; **277**: 909–914.

American Academy of Pediatrics v. Heckler, 561. F. Suppl. 395 (DDC 1983).

Anand KJS, Sippell WG, Aynsley-Green A. Randomised trial of fentanyl anaesthesia in preterm babies undergoing surgery: effects of the stress response. *Lancet* 1987a; **i**: 62–66.

Anand KJS, Hickey PR. Pain and its effects in the human neonate and fetus. *New England Journal of Medicine* 1987b; **317**: 1321–1329.

Anand KJS, Hansen DD, Hickey PR. Hormonal-metabolic stress responses in neonates undergoing cardiac surgery. *Anaesthesiology* 1990; **73**: 661–670.

Anand KJS, Hickey PR. Halothane-morphine compared with high-dose fentanyl for anaesthesia and post-operative analgesia in neonatal cardiac surgery. *New England Journal of Medicine* 1992; **326**: 1–9.

Annas GJ. *Judging Medicine*. Clifton, New Jersey: Humana Press, 1988.

Annas GJ. Asking the courts to set the standard of emergency care—the case of Baby K. *New England Journal of Medicine* 1994; **330**: 1542–1545.

Annas GJ. quoted in Miller FG, Fins JJ. Sounding board. A proposal to restructure hospital care for dying patients. *New England Journal of Medicine* 1996; **334**: 1740–1742.

Annotation. Cardiac resuscitation in hospital: more restraint needed! *Lancet* 1982; **i**: 27–28.

Annotation. Infant mortality. *Lancet* 1988; **ii**: 1117–1118.

Anonymous. Who and what. *Pediatrics* 1975; **55**: 753–755.

Apgar V. A proposal for a new method of evaluation of the newborn infant. *Anaesthesia and Analgesia* 1953; **32**: 260–267.

Applebaum PS, Lidz CW, Meisel A. *Informed Consent. Legal Theory and Clinical Practice*. New York: Oxford University Press, 1987.

Armitage P. Bradford Hill and the randomized controlled trial. *Pharmaceutical Medicine* 1992; **6**: 23–37.

Armstrong JS. Peer review of scientific papers. *Journal of Biological Response Modifiers* 1984; **3**: 10–14.

Asher R. Sense and Sensibility. The Lettsomian Lectures for 1959. *Transactions of the Medical Society of London* 1958–59; **75**: 66–72.

Asher R. *Talking Sense*. Tunbridge Wells: Pittman Medical Publications, 1972.

Associated Press. Doctor who euthanizes baby off the hook. April 28, 1995.

Bacon F. In: Fowler T. (editor) *Novum Organum*. Oxford: Clarendon Press, 1878.

Bailar JC. III. Research quality, methodologic rigor, citation counts, and impact. *American Journal of Public Health* 1982; **72**: 1103–1104.

Bailar JC III. When research results are in conflict. *New England Journal of Medicine* 1985; **b 313**: 1080–1081.

Bailar JC III, Paterson K. Journal peer review. The need for a research agenda. *New England Journal of Medicine* 1985; **a 312**: 654–657.

Balint M. *The Doctor, His Patient and the Illness*. New York: International University Press, 1957.

Ballantyne JW. The problem of the premature infant. *British Medical Journal* 1902; **i**: 1106–1110.

Bartholome WG. A new understanding of consent in pediatric practice. *Pediatric Annals* 1989; **18**: 262–265.

Bartlett RH, Gazzaniga AB, Jeffries MR *et al*. Extracorporeal membrane oxygenation (ECMO) cardiopulmonary support in infancy. *Transactions of the American Society of Artificial Organs* 1976; **22**: 80–93.

Bartlett RH, Roloff DW, Cornell RG *et al*. Extracorporeal circulation in neonatal respiratory failure. A prospective randomized study. *Pediatrics* 1985; **76**: 479–487.

Bascom WR (compiler). *African Dilemma Tales*. The Hague: Mouton Publishers, 1975. (Note Bascom's version appears on p. 94 and is derived from the tale recorded by Trautmann R. La Littérature Populair à côte des Esclaves. *Travaux et Mémoires de l'Institut d'Ethnologie* IV, 1927. Institut d'Ethnologie, Paris 1927.)

Bates EM. The implications for semantics for developments in medical technology and the fatal consequences of semantic ignorance. *Et Cetera* 1980; **10**: 25–32.

Bearman JE, Loewenson RB, Gullen WH. Muench's postulates, laws and corollaries. *Biometrics Notes*, Number 4, National Eye Institute, 1974.

Beauchamp TL, Childress JF. *Principles in Biomedical Ethics.* New York: Oxford University Press, 1979.

Becker LB, Han BH, Meyer PM et al. Racial differences in the incidence of cardiac arrest and subsequent survival. *New England Journal of Medicine* 1993; **329**: 600–606.

Beecher HK. Ethics and clinical research. *New England Journal of Medicine* 1966; **274**: 1354–1360.

Begg C, Cho M, Eastwood S et al. Improving the quality of reporting of randomized controlled trials. The CONSORT Statement. *Journal of the American Medical Association* 1996; **276**: 637–639.

Bell R. The Cantekin dispute and the Bluestone case. In: Bell R (editor). *Impure Science.* New York: John Wiley, 1992.

Berendes HW. The structure and scope of the Collaborative Project on Cerebral Palsy, Mental Retardation, and other Neurological and Sensory Disorders of Infancy and Childhood. In: Chipman SS, Lilienfeld AM, Greenberg BG et al. (editors). *Research Methodology and Needs in Perinatal Studies.* Springfield, Illinois: Charles Thomas, 1966.

Bernier CL, Yerkey AN. *Cogent Communication: Overcoming Reading Overload.* Westport, Connecticut: Greenwood Publishers, 1979.

Bifano EM, Hakanson DO, Hingre RV et al. Prospective randomized controlled trial of conventional treatment or transport for ECMO in infants with persistent pulmonary hypertension (PPHN). *Pediatric Research* 1992; **31**: 196A (Abstract).

Blair E, Stanley FJ. Intrapartum asphyxia: a rare cause of cerebral palsy. *Journal of Pediatrics* 1988; **112**: 515–519.

Blair VP. Some notes on the care of premature infants. *St Louis Medical Review* 1904; **49**: 321–324.

Blendon RJ, Szalay US, Knox RA. Should physicians aid their patients in dying? The public perspective. *Journal of the American Medical Association* 1992; **267**: 2658–2662.

Bloom BS. Changing infant mortality: the need to spend more while getting less. *Pediatrics* 1986; **73**: 862–866.

Blum AL, Chalmers TC, Deutsch J et al. Lugano statement on controlled clinical trials. *Journal of International Research* 1987; **15**: 2–22.

Boorstin DJ. *Cleopatra's Nose. Essays on the Unexpected.* New York: Random House, 1994.

Boston Interhospital Virus Study Group. Delaying double-blind drug evaluation in usually fatal diseases (letter). *New England Journal of Medicine* 1975; **293**: 509.

Boston Women's Health Book Collective. *Our Bodies, Ourselves: A Book By and For Women.* New York: Simon and Schuster, 1971.

Botkin JR. Delivery room decisions for tiny infants: an ethical analysis. *Journal of Clinical Ethics* 1990; **1**: 306–311.

Boyle MH., Torrance GW, Sinclair JC *et al*. Economic evaluation of neonatal intensive care of very-low-birth-weight infants. *New England Journal of Medicine* 1983; **308**: 1330–1337.

Bracken MB. Clinical trials and the acceptance of uncertainty. *British Medical Journal* 1987; **294**: 1111–1112.

Braff J. Parallel track (letter). *New York Times* December 20, 1989.

Braine Sir B. Medicine and the media. MP apologises. *British Medical Journal* 1988; **297**: 865.

Bray J. Health care: One product's story. *New York Times* January 15, 1995.

Bray J. Trouble in the waiting line for heart transplants. *New York Times* January 26, 1997.

Brewin CR, Bradley C. Patient preferences and randomised clinical trials. *British Journal of Medicine* 1989; **299**: 313–315.

Brody H. Transparency: informed consent in primary care. *Hastings Center Report* 1989; **19**: 5–9.

Brody H. *The Healer's Power*. New Haven: Yale University Press, 1992.

Brody H. *Ethical Issues in Drug Testing, Approval, and Pricing. The Clot-Dissolving Drugs*. Oxford: Oxford University Press, 1996.

Bruer JT. Methodological rigor and citation frequency in patient compliance literature. *American Journal of Public Health* 1982; **72**: 1119–1122.

Buchanan N. The very-low-birthweight infant—medical, ethical, legal and economic considerations. *Medical Journal of Australia* 1987; **147**: 184–186.

Buck v. Bell. Supreme Court Reporter (274 U.S. 200), 1927.

Budin P. *The Nursling*. (Translated by WJ Maloney). London: The Caxton Publishing Company, 1907.

Burman KD. Hanging from the masthead: reflections on authorship. *Annals of Internal Medicine* 1982; **97**: 602–605.

Burroughs J. *Indoor Studies*. New York: Houghton Mifflin Company, 1900.

Cahn E. Drug experiments and the public conscience. In: Katz J (editor). *Experimentation with Human Beings*. New York: Russell Sage Foundation, 1972.

Callahan D. *What Kind of Life? The Limits of Medical Progress*. New York: Simon and Schuster, 1990.

Callahan D. *The Troubled Dream of Life*. New York: Simon and Schuster, 1993.

Callahan D. Bioethics: private choice and the common good. *Hastings Center Report* 1994; **24**: 28–31.

Campbell AGM. Commentary. *Archives of Disease in Childhood* 1988; **63**: 565–566.

Campion EW. Why unconventional medicine? *New England Journal of Medicine* 1993; **328**: 282–283.

Candee D, Sheehan TJ, Cook CD *et al*. Moral reasoning in dilemmas of neonatal care. *Pediatric Research* 1982; **16**: 846–850.

Cantekin EI, McGuire TW, Potter RL. Biomedical information, peer review, and conflict of interest as they influence public health. *Journal of the American Medical Association* 1990; **263**: 1427–1430.

Cantekin EI, McGuire TW, Griffith TL. Antimicrobial therapy for otitis media with effusion ('secretory' otitis media). *Journal of the American Medical Association* 1991; **266**: 3309–3317.

Cardiac Arrhythmia Suppression Trial (CAST) Investigators. Preliminary report: Increased mortality due to encainide or flecainide in a randomized trial of arrhythmia suppression after myocardial infarction. *New England Journal of Medicine* 1989; **321**: 406–412.

Cardiac Arrhythmia Suppression Trial (CAST II) Investigators. Effect of the anti-arrhythmic agent moricizine on survival after myocardial infarction. *New England Journal of Medicine* 1992; **327**: 227–233.

Cassileth BR, Lusk EJ, Miller MA *et al.* Attitudes toward clinical trials among patients and the public. *Journal of the American Medical Association* 1982; **248**: 968–970.

Castiglioni A. *A History of Medicine.* New York: Knopf, 1941.

Chalmers I, Silverman WA. Professional and public double-standards on clinical experimentation. *Controlled Clinical Trials* 1987; **8**: 388–391.

Chalmers I, Enkin M, Kierse MJNC (editors). *Effective Care in Pregnancy and Child-birth.* Oxford: Oxford University Press, 1989.

Chalmers I, Dickersin K, Chalmers TC. Getting to grips with Archie Cochrane's agenda. All randomised controlled trials should be registered. *British Medical Journal* 1992; **305**: 786–788.

Chalmers TC, Block, JB, Lee S. Controlled studies in clinical cancer research. *New England Journal of Medicine* 1972; **287**: 75–78.

Chapin HD. The rearing of premature infants by means of incubators. *Archives of Pediatrics* 1900; **17**: 37–39.

Churchill LR. Bioethical reductionism and our sense of the human. *Man and Medicine* 1980; **5**: 229–242.

Churchill LR. *Self-Interest and Universal Health Care.* Cambridge, Massachusetts: Harvard University Press, 1994.

Churchill LR, King NMP. Physician assisted suicide, euthanasia, or withdrawal of treatment. *British Medical Journal* 1997; **315**: 137–138.

Claiborne W. Paralyzed Canadian woman wins court approval ruling on right to die. *Washington Post* January 7, 1992.

Clark FI. Making sense of State v. Messenger. *Pediatrics* 1996; **97**: 579–583.

Clausewitz von, K. *Vom Kriege.* Memorial Edition, 1952.

Cobb LA, Thomas GI, Dillard DH *et al.* An evaluation of internal-mammary-artery ligation by a double-blind technic. *New England Journal of Medicine* 1959; **260**: 1115–1118.

Cochrane AL. *Effectiveness and Efficiency. Random Reflections on Health Services.* London: Nuffield Provincial Hospitals Trust, 1972.

Cochrane AL. 1931–1971: a critical review with particular reference to the medical profession. In *Medicines for the Year 2000.* London: Office of Health Economics, 1979.

Cohen CB, Levin B, Powderly K. Section I: a history of neonatal intensive care and decision-making. *Hastings Center Report* 1987; **17**: 7–9.

Cohen IB. *Revolution in Science.* Cambridge, Massachusetts: Belknap Press, 1985.

Cohen MM, Weintraub D, Lilienfeld AM. The relationship of pulmonary hyaline membranes to certain factors in pregnancy and delivery. *Pediatrics* 1960; **26**: 42–50.

Comment. Matters of life and death. *The Guardian* November 15, 1981.

Comroe JH Jr. *Retrospectroscope. Insights Into Medical Discovery.* Menlo Park, California: Von Gehr Press, 1977.

Cone TE Jr. *History of the Care and Feeding of the Premature Infant.* Boston: Little, Brown, 1985.

Connors AF, Speroff T, Dawson NV *et al*. The effectiveness of right heart catheterization in the initial care of critically ill patients. *Journal of the American Medical Association* 1996; **276**: 889–897.

Cook DJ, Guyatt GH, Jaeschke R *et al*. Determinants in Canadian health care workers of the decision to withdraw life support. *Journal of the Canadian Medical Association* 1995; **273**: 703–709.

Cook RJ, Sackett DL. The number needed to treat: A clinically useful measure of the treatment effect. *British Medical Journal* 1995; **310**: 452–454.

Counsell CE, Sandercock PAG. Failure to publish completed randomised controlled trials is unethical in itself (letter). *British Medical Journal* 1997; **314**: 1481.

Crosse VM. *The Premature Baby*. London: Churchill, Livingstone, 1945.

Cryotherapy for Retinopathy of Prematurity Cooperative Group. Multicenter trial of cryotherapy for retinopathy of prematurity: preliminary results. *Pediatrics* 1988; **81**: 697–706.

Cryotherapy for Retinopathy of Prematurity Cooperative Group. Multicenter trial of cryotherapy for retinopathy of prematurity: 3½-year outcome—structure and function. *Archives of Ophthalmology* 1993; **111**: 339–344.

Cryotherapy for Retinopathy of Prematurity Cooperative Group. Multicenter trial of cryotherapy for retinopathy of prematurity: Snellen visual acuity and structural outcome at 5½-years. *Archives of Ophthalmology* 1996; **114**: 417–424.

Daily Mail (UK) July 8, 1987.

Dancis J. *Idiopathic Respiratory Distress Syndrome* [Proceeding of the interdisciplinary conferences in 1967 and 1968]. Bethesda: US Public Health Service/National Institutes of Health, 1968.

Darnton R. *Mesmerism and the End of the Enlightenment in France*. Cambridge, Massachusetts: Harvard University Press, 1968.

Darwin C, Wallace ARW. On the tendency of species to form varieties; and on the perpetuation of varieties by natural means of selection. *Journal of the Linnaean Society of London (Zoology)* 1858; **3**: 45–62.

Davis JM, Spitzer AR, Cox C et al. Predicting survival in infants with persistent pulmonary hypertension of the newborn. *Paediatric Pulmonology* 1988; **5**: 6–9.

Deber RB, Thompson GG. Variations in breast cancer treatment decisions and their impact in mounting trials. *Controlled Clinical Trials* 1990; **11**: 353–373.

Department of Health and Human Services. Nondiscrimination on the basis of handicap relating to health care for handicapped infants. *Federal Register* 1984; **49** 1622–1654.

Descartes R. *Discourse on Method* (Translated by L.J. Lafleur). Indianapolis: Bobbs-Merill, 1956.

Dieckman WJ, Davis ME, Rynkiewicz LM *et al*. Does the administration of diethylstilbestrol during pregnancy have therapeutic values? American *Journal of Obstetrics and Gynecology* 1953; **66**: 1062–1081.

Doe (In re), Circuit Court for Monroe County. Indiana, No. GU 8204–004A, order signed April 12, 1982.

Doxiadis S. Introduction. In: Doxiadis S (editor). *Ethical Dilemmas in Health Care Promotion*. Chichester: John Wiley & Sons, 1987.

Dreyfuss R. Popping contributions. The new battle for the FDA. *American Prospect* 1997; **33** (July–August): 53–58.

Drummond JC, Wilbraham A. *The Englishman's Food: A History of Five Centuries*. London: Jonathan Cape, 1940.

Dubos R. *Mirage of Health: Utopias, Progress and Equality.* New York: Harper Colophon Books, 1979.

Duc G, Sinclair JC. Oxygen administration. In: Sinclair JC, Bracken MB (editors). *Effective Care of the Newborn Infant.* Oxford: Oxford University Press, 1992a.

Duc G, Sinclair JC. Oxygen administration. In: Sinclair JC, Bracken MB (editors). *Effective Care of the Newborn.* Oxford: Oxford University Press, 1992b.

Dudley HAF. Extracranial-intracranial bypass, one; clinical trials, nil. *British Medical Journal* 1987; **294**: 1501–1502.

Durack DT. The weight of medical knowledge. *New England Journal of Medicine* 1978; **298**: 773–775.

Dworetz AR, Moya FR, Sabo B *et al.* Survival of infants with persistent pulmonary hypertension without extracorporeal membrane oxygenation. *Pediatrics* 1989; **84**: 1–6.

Dworkin R. *Taking Rights Seriously.* Cambridge, Massachusetts: Harvard University Press, 1991.

Dworkin R. *Life's Dominion.* New York: Knopf, 1993.

Dworkin R. Will Clinton's plan be fair? *New York Review of Books* January 13, 1994.

Dyson F. Reflections. *New Yorker Magazine* February 6, 1984.

Eddy DM. Clinical decision-making: from theory to practice. *Journal of the American Medical Association* 1990; **263**: 283–290, 877–880, 1265–1275, 1839–1841.

Ederer F. Patient bias, investigator bias and the double-masked procedure in clinical trials. *American Journal of Medicine* 1975; **58**: 295–299.

Editorial. Pain, anaesthesia, and babies. *Lancet* 1987; **ii**: 543–544.

Editorial. Limitations of care for very-low-birthweight infants. *Lancet* 1988; **i**: 1257–1258.

Editorial. Compassionate release of DDI. *Lancet* 1989; **ii**: 1079–1080.

Editorial. Cochrane's legacy. *Lancet* 1992; **340**: 1131–1132.

Editorial. Time for education in palliative care. *Lancet* 1997; **349**: 1709.

Editorial board. Point-counterpoint. Physicians' refusal of requested treatment. *Journal of Perinatology* 1990; **10**: 407–415.

Edlund MJ, Craig TJ, Richardson MA. Informed consent as a form of volunteer bias. *American Journal of Psychiatry* 1985; **142**: 624–627.

Eisenberg DM, Kessler RC, Foster C *et al.* Unconventional medicine in the United States. Prevalence, costs and patterns of use. *New England Journal of Medicine* 1993; **328**: 246–252.

Eisenberg L. From circumstances to mechanism in pediatrics during the Hopkins Century. *Pediatrics* 1990; **85**: 42–49.

Ellenberg JH. Cohort studies. Selection bias in observational and experimental studies. *Statistics in Medicine* 1994; **13**: 557–567.

Elliott SJ. Neonatal extracorporeal membrane oxygenation: how not to assess novel technologies. *Lancet* 1991; **337**: 476–477.

Ellul J. An ethics of nonpower (translated by Levy NK). In: Kranz J, Berg M (editors). *Ethics in an Age of Pervasive Technology.* Boulder, Colorado: Westview Press, 1980.

Emery JL. Attitudes of parents and paediatricians to a baby's death. *Journal of the Royal Society of Medicine* 1990; **83**: 423–424.

Engelhardt HT Jr. Bioethics in pluralist societies. *Perspectives in Biology and Medicine* 1982; **26**: 64–78.

Epstein E, Pinski JB. A blind study. *Archives of Dermatology* 1961; **89**: 548–549.

Ertl N. A new way of documenting scientific data from medical publications. *Karger Gazette* 1969; **20** (November 27): 1–3.

Escobar GJ, Littenberg B, Petitti DF. Outcome among surviving very low birth-weight infants: a meta-analysis. *Archives of Disease in Childhood* 1991; **66**: 204–211.

Etzel RA, Pattishall EN, Haley NH *et al.* Passive smoking and middle ear effusion among children in day care. *Pediatrics* 1992; **90**: 228–232.

Etzioni A. The responsive community (I and we). *American Sociologist* 1987; **18**: 146–150.

Excerpts. The decision in 'Baby Jane Doe' case. *New York Times* October 29, 1981.

Faden RR, Beauchamp TL. *A History and Theory of Informed Consent.* New York: Oxford University Press, 1986.

Fahey T, Griffiths S, Peters TJ. Evidence based purchasing: understanding results of clinical trials and systematic reviews. *British Journal of Medicine* 1995; **311**: 1056–1059.

FDA. *General Considerations for the Clinical Evaluation of Drugs.* HEW Publication No.(FDA) 77–3040, Washington, DC, 1977.

Feinstein A R. Invidious comparisons and unmet clinical challenges. *American Journal of Medicine* 1992; **92**: 117–120.

Ferriman A. Wide support for Down's doctor. *The Times* November 10, 1981.

Fetus and Newborn Committee of the American Academy of Pediatrics. Recommendation on extracorporeal membrane oxygenation. *Pediatrics* 1990; **85**: 618–619.

Fetus and Newborn Committee of the American Academy of Pediatrics; Committee on Obstetric Practice of the American College of Obstetrics and Gynecologists. Perinatal Care at the Threshold of Viability. *Pediatrics* 1995; **96**: 974–976.

Fetus and Newborn Committee of the Canadian Pediatric Society. *Statement: Approach to the Women with Threatened Birth of an Extremely Low Gestational Age Infant (22–26 completed weeks).* Ottawa, Ontario: Canadian Pediatric Society Secretariat October 1993.

Fetus and Newborn Committee of the Canadian Pediatric Society and Maternal-Fetal Medicine Committee, Society of Obstetricians and Gynecologists of Canada. Management of the woman with threatened birth of an extremely low gestational age. *Canadian Medical Association Journal* 1994; **151**: 547–553.

Final Report of the Dutch State Commission on Euthanasia (English translation). *Bioethics* 1987; **1**: 163–174.

Findley T. The placebo and the physician. *Medical Clinics of North America* 1953; **37**: 1821–1826.

First (The) International Congress on Peer Review. Guarding the Guardians: Research on Peer Review. *Journal of the American Medical Association* 1989; **263**: 1317–1408.

Fisher RA. The arrangements of field experiments. *Journal of the Ministry of Agriculture* 1926; **33**: 503–506.

Fisher RA. Quoted in Mainland D. The use and misuse of statistics in medical publications. *Clinical Pharmacological Therapy* 1960; **1**: 411–412.

Fleischman AR. Overtreatment of neonates (letter). *Pediatrics* 1993; **263**: 169–171.

Fleischman AR. Physicians' refusal of requested treatment: views from the Journal's editorial board. *Journal of Perinatology* 1990; **10**: 407–415.

Fletcher W. Rice and beri-beri; Preliminary report on an experiment conducted at the Kuala Lumpur Lunatic Asylum. *Lancet* 1907; **i**: 1776–1779.

Forfar JO, Campbell AGM. Medicine and the media. *British Medical Journal* 1987; **295**: 659–660.

Foster C. Why do research ethics committees disagree with each other? *Journal of the Royal College of Physicians* 1995; **29**: 315–318.

Fox RC, Swazey JP. Leaving the field. *Hastings Center Report* 1992a; **September–October**: 9–15.

Fox RC, Swazey JP. *Spare Parts.* Oxford: Oxford University Press, 1992b.

Frankel MS. The development of policy guidelines governing human experimentation in the United States: A case study of public policy-making for science and technology. *Ethics in Science and Medicine* 1975; **2**: 43–59.

Freedman B. Equipoise and the ethics of clinical research. *New England Journal of Medicine* 1987; **317**: 141–145.

Freidson E. *Profession of Medicine. A Study of the Sociology of Applied Knowledge.* New York: Dodd Mead, 1972.

Freirich EJ, Gehan EA. The limitations of the randomized clinical trial. In: DeVita VT Jr, Busch H (editors). *Methods in Cancer Research. Volume XVII. Cancer Drug Development Part B.* London: Academic Press, 1979.

Fried C. *Medical Experimentation: Personal Integrity and Social Policy.* Amsterdam: North Holland Publishing Company, 1974.

Frohock FM. *Special Care: Medical Decisions at the Beginning of Life.* Chicago: University of Chicago Press, 1986.

Galbraith JK. *The Age of Uncertainty.* Boston: Houghton Mifflin, 1977.

Galton F. Statistical inquiries into the efficacy of prayer. *Fortnightly Review* August 1, 1872.

Gardner MJ, Altman DG. Confidence intervals rather than P values: estimation rather than hypothesis testing. *British Medical Journal* 1986; **292**: 746–750.

Georgescu-Roegen N. Utility and value in economic thought. In: Weinert PP (editor). *Dictionary of Ideas.* New York: Charles Scribner's Sons, 1974.

Gerry MH, Nimz M. The federal role in protecting Babies Doe. *Issues in Law and Medicine* 1987; **2**: 239–377.

Gifford F. The conflict between randomized clinical trials and the therapeutic obligation. *Journal of Medicine and Philosophy* 1986; **11**: 347–366.

Gilbert C, Rahi, J, Eckstein M et al. Retinopathy of prematurity in middle-income countries. *Lancet* 1997; **350**: 12–14.

Goldsmith O. *The Bee,* 1759.

Goldstein PA, Sacks HS, Chalmers TC. Chapter 38. Hormone administration for the maintenance of pregnancy. In: Chalmers I, Enkin M, Keirse MJN (editors). *Effective Care in Pregnancy and Childbirth.* Oxford: Oxford University Press, 1989.

Goldworth A, Benitz WE. The case of Baby L revisted. *Clinical Pediatrics* 1995; **34**: 452–456.

Gøtzsche PC. Methodology and overt and hidden bias in reports of 196 double-blind trials of nonsteroidal anti-inflammatory drugs in rheumatoid arthritis. *Controlled Clinical Trials* 1989; 10: 31–56. Correction 1989; **10**: 356.

Gould SJ. The chain of reason versus the chain of thumbs. In: Gould SJ (editor). *Bully for Brontosaurus.* New York: W.W. Norton & Company, 1991.

Grace ND, Muench H, Chalmers TC. The present status of shunts for portal hypertension in cirrhosis. *Gastroenterology* 1966; **50**: 684–691.

Greenberg RP, Fisher S. Seeing through the double-mask design: a commentary. *Controlled Clinical Trials* 1994; **15**: 244–246.

Greer AL. Diffusion of medical technology. The case of ECMO. In: Wright L (editor). *Report of a Workshop on Diffusion of ECMO Technology.* Bethesda, Maryland: National Institute of Technology Publication No. 93–3399; 1993.

Greer AL. Scientific knowledge and social consensus. *Controlled Clinical Trials* 1994; **15**: 431–436.

Gribben M. Placebos: Cheapest medicine in the world. *New Scientist* 1981; **89**: 64–65.

Guillemin J. An exchange on Baby Doe. *New York Review of Books.* June 14, 1984.

Guillemin JH, Holmstrom LL. *Mixed Blessings. Intensive Care for Newborns.* Oxford: Oxford University Press, 1986.

Gustaitis, R, Young EWD. *A Time to be Born. A Time to Die.* Reading, Massachusetts: Addison Wesley, 1986.

Guyatt GH. Evidence-based medicine. *Annals of Internal Medicine* 1991; **114** (American College of Physicians Journal Club Supplement 2): A16.

Guyatt GH, Sackett DL, Sinclair JC *et al.* Users' guides to the medical literature. IX A method for grading health care recommendations. *Journal of the American Medical Association* 1995; **274**: 1800–1804.

Guyer B, Strobino DM, Ventura SJ *et al.* Annual summary of vital statistics. *Pediatrics* 1994; **96**: 1029–1034.

Hack M, Fanaroff AA. Outcome of extremely-low-birth-weight infants between 1982 and 1988. *New England Journal of Medicine* 1989; **321**: 1642–1647.

Hack M, Fanaroff AA. Outcomes of extremely immature infants—a perinatal dilemma. *New England Journal of Medicine* 1993; **329**: 1649–1650.

Haines A, Jones R. Implementing findings of research. *British Medical Journal* 1994; **308**: 1488–1492.

Hall SS. *A Commotion in the Blood.* New York: Henry Holt, 1997.

Hallman M. Bry K, Hoppu K *et al.* Inositol supplementation in premature infants with respiratory distress syndrome. *New England Journal of Medicine* 1992; **326**: 1233–1239.

Hardwick M, Hardwick M. *The Man Who was Sherlock Holmes.* New York: Doubleday, 1964.

Harrison H. The principles for family-centered neonatal care. *Pediatrics* 1993; **92**: 643–650.

Harrison H. Commentary. The Messenger case. *Journal of Perinatology* 1996; **16**: 299–301.

Harth SC, Thong YH. Sociodemographic and motivational characteristics of parents who volunteer their children for clinical research: a controlled study. *British Medical Journal* 1990; **300**: 1372–1375.

Hayek FA. *The Constitution of Liberty.* Chicago: University of Chicago Press, 1960.

Haygarth J. *Of the Imagination, as a Cause and Cure of Disorders of the Body: Exemplified by Fictitious Tractors and Epidemical Convulsions.* Bath: R Crutwell, 1800.

Haynes RB, Mulrow CD, Huth EJ *et al.* More informative abstracts revisited. *Annals of Internal Medicine* 1990; **113**: 69–76.

Healy JB. Why do you write? (letter) *Lancet* 1976; **i**: 204.

Healy MJR. Is statistics a science? *Journal of the Royal Statistical Society,* Series A 1978; **141**: 385–393.

Heide van der A, van der Maas PJ, van der Wal G *et al.* Medical end-of-life decisions made for neonates and infants in the Netherlands. *Lancet* 1997; **350**: 251–255.

Henaean J. Eighty per cent of preemies in follow-up essentially normal by age two. *Medical Tribune* 1979; **20**: 1–20.

Hendin H. *Seduced by Death. Doctors, Patients and the Dutch Cure.* New York: WW Norton, 1997.

Henshaw RC, Naji SA, Russell IT *et al.* Comparison of medical abortion with surgical vacuum aspiration: women's preferences. *British Medical Journal* 1993; **307**: 714–717.

Herbst AL, Ulfelder H, Poskanzer DC. Adenocarcinoma of the vagina: Association of maternal stilbestrol therapy with tumor appearance in young women. *New England Journal of Medicine* 1971; **284**: 878–891.

Hershey CO, Fisher L. Why outcome of cardiopulmonary resuscitation in general wards is poor. *Lancet* 1982; **i**: 31–34.

Hey E. Retrolental fibroplasia as one index of perinatally acquired handicap. In: Chalmers I, McIllwaine G (editors). *Perinatal Audit and Surveillance.* London: Royal College of Obstetrics and Gynaecology, 1980.

Hilgard EL. Introduction. In: Mesmer FA (Translated by GJ Bloch). *Mesmerism.* Los Altos, California: William Kaufman, 1980.

Hill AB. *Principles of Medical Statistics.* Oxford: Oxford University Press, 1937.

Hill AB. The philosophy of the clinical trial. In: Hill AB (editor). *Statistical Methods in Clinical and Preventive Medicine.* London: E&S Livingstone, 1962.

Hill Sir AB. Memories of the British streptomycin trial in tuberculosis. *Controlled Clinical Trials* 1990;11: 77–79.

Hofstadter R. *Social Darwinism in American Thought.* Boston: Beacon Press, 1955.

Holder AR. Parents, courts, and refusal of treatment. *Journal of Pediatrics* 1983; **103**: 515–521.

Holmes OW, quoted in Gaylin W, Jennings B. *The Perversion of Autonomy.* New York: Free Press, 1996.

Horbar JD, Badger GJ, Lewit EM *et al.* Hospital and patient characteristics associated with variation in 28-day mortality rates for very low birth weight infants. *Pediatrics* 1997; **99**: 149–156.

Horton R. Pardonable revisions and protocol reviews. *Lancet* 1997; **349**: 6.

Houston WR. The doctor himself as therapeutic agent. *Annals of Internal Medicine* 1938; **11**: 416–420.

Hughes EC. *Men and Their Work.* New York: Free Press, 1958.

Hull D. The viable child. The Croonian Lecture 1988. *Journal of the Royal College of Physicians of London* 1988; **2**: 169–175.

Hume D. *A Treatise of Human Nature,* 2nd edition. In: Selby-Bigge LA, Nidditch PH (editors). Oxford: Clarendon Press, 1978.

Hutchison GB. Discussion of Weiss W. The analysis of data in the collaborative project of the National Institute of Neurological Disease and Blindness. In: Chipman SS, Lilienfeld AM, Greenberg BG *et al.* (editors). *Research Methodology and Needs in Perinatal Studies.* Springfield, Illinois: Charles C. Thomas, 1966.

Huth EJ. Structured abstracts for papers reporting clinical trials (Editorial). *Annals of Internal Medicine* 1987; **106**: 626–627.

Infant Bioethics Task Force. Guidelines for infant bioethics committees. *Pediatrics* 1984; **74**: 306–310.

Insight Team of the *Sunday Times* of London. *Suffer the Children. The Story of Thalidomide.* New York: Viking, 1979.

Institute of Medicine. *Vitamin E and Retinopathy of Prematurity.* Washington, DC: National Academy Press (June), 1986.

Institute of Medicine. *Approaching Death: Improving Care at the End Of Life.* Washington, DC: National Academy Press (June), 1997.

Jameton AL. Paediatric nursing ethics. In: Goldworth A, Silverman W, Stevenson DK *et al.* (editors). *Ethics and Perinatology.* Oxford: Oxford University Press, 1995.

Janis IL, Mann L. *Decision Making. A Psychological Analysis of Conflict, Choice, and Committment.* London: Collier Macmillan Publishers, 1977.

Jennett B. Assessment of a technology package using a predictive tool. *International Journal of Technological Assessment in Health Care* 1987; **3**: 335–338.

Johansson J-E, Holmberg L, Johansson S *et al.* Fifteen-year survival in prostate cancer. A prospective, population-based study. *Journal of the American Medical Association* 1997; **277**: 467–471.

Jolley D. The glitter of the *t* table. *Lancet* 1993; **342**: 27–29.

Jonas H. Philosophical reflections on experimenting with human subjects. *Daedalus* 1969; **219**: 223–245.

Jonas H. *The Imperative of Responsibility. In Search for an Ethics for the Technological Age.* Chicago: University of Chicago Press, 1984.

Judson HF. Structural transformations of the sciences and the end of peer review. *Journal of the American Medical Association* 1994; **272**: 92–94.

Kanto WP. A decade of experience with neonatal extracorporeal membrane oxygenation. *Journal of Pediatrics* 1994; **124**: 335–347.

Katz J. *Experimentation with Human Beings.* New York: Russell Sage Foundation, 1972.

Katz J. *The Silent World of Doctor and Patient.* New York: Free Press, 1984.

Kavanaugh C, Sorenson JR, Swazey JP. We shall overcome: Multi-institutional review of a genetic counseling study. *IRB: A Review of Human Subjects Research* 1979; **1**: 1–3.

Kelsey FO. Government: The Kefauver-Harris Amendments and investigational drugs. *American Journal of Hospital Pharmacy* 1963; **20**: 515–517.

Kidder RM. *How Good People Make Tough Choices.* New York: William Morrow, 1995.

Kimbrell A. *The Human Body Shop.* New York: Harper Collins, 1993.

King NMP. Transparency in neonatal intensive care. *Hastings Center Report* 1992; **22**: 18–25.

Kinsey VE. Etiology of retrolental fibroplasia and preliminary report of the Co-operative Study of Retrolental Fibroplasia. *Transactions of the American Academy of Ophthalmology* 1955; **59**: 15–24.

Knox RA. A Harvard study on newborns draws fire: doctor faulted for limiting life-saving therapy. *Boston Globe* August 7, 1989.

Kohlberg L. Moral stages and moralization: the cognitive-developmental approach. In: Likona T (editor). *Moral Development and Behavior.* New York: Holt, Rinehart and Wilson, 1976.

Kolata G. Innovative AIDS drug plan may be undermining testing. *New York Times* November 21, 1989.

Kolata G. Study finds 2-decade decline in sperm counts in fertile men. *New York Times* February 2, 1995.

Kolata G. Lack of volunteers thwarts research on prostate cancer. *New York Times* February 12, 1997.

Kolata G. Scientist reports first cloning ever of adult mammal. *New York Times* February 23, 1997.

Konner M. *The Tangled Wing*. New York: Holt, Rinehart and Wilson, 1982.

Konner M. *Becoming a Doctor. A Journey of Initiation in Medical School*. New York: Viking, 1987.

Kopelman LM, Irons TG, Kopelman AE. Neonatologists judge the 'Baby Doe' regulations. *New England Journal of Medicine* 1988; **318**: 677–683.

Korn EL, Baumrind S. Randomised clinical trials with clinician-preferred treatment. *Lancet* 1991; **337**: 149–152.

Koshland D Jr. Editorial: The golden mean. *Science* 1988; **242**: 1255.

Kuban KCK, Leviton A, Krishnamoorthy KS *et al*. Neonatal intracranial hemorrhage and phenobarbital. *Pediatrics* 1988; **77**: 443–450.

Kuhn TS. *The Structure of Scientific Revolutions*. Chicago: University of Chicago Press, 1970.

Kulkarni P, Hall RT, Rhodes PG *et al*. Postneonatal mortality in infants admitted to a neonatal intensive care unit. *Pediatrics* 1978; **62**: 178–183.

Ladimer I. Ethical and legal aspects of medical research on human beings. In: Ladimer I, Newman R (editors). *Clinical Investigations in Medicine*. Boston: University Law-Medicine Institute, 1963.

Lakatos L, Oroszlan G. Possible effect of D-penicillamine on the physiological action of inhaled nitric oxide in neonates (letter). *Journal of Pediatrics* 1994; **124**: 656–657.

Lakatos L, Hatvani I, Oroszlan G *et al*. Prevention of retrolental fibroplasia in very low birth weight infants by d-penicillamine. *European Journal of Pediatrics* 1982; **138**: 199–200.

Lakatos L, Hatvani I Oroszlan G *et al*. Controlled trial of d-penicillamine to prevent retinopathy of prematurity. *Acta Paediatrica Hungarica* 1986; **27**: 47–56.

Lamm RD. The ethics of excess. *Hastings Center Report* 1994; **24**: 14.

Lantos JD, Frader J. Sounding board: Extracorporeal membrane oxygenation and the ethics of clinical research. *New England Journal of Medicine* 1990; **323**: 409–413.

Larson ML. *The Rise of Professionalism. A Sociological Analysis*. Berkeley: University of California Press, 1978.

Lasagna L. The diseases drugs cause. *Perspectives in Biology and Medicine* 1964; **Summer**: 457–470.

Last JM (editor). *A Dictionary of Epidemiology*. Oxford: Oxford University Press, 1983.

Lawson JR. Letter to the Editor. *Birth* 1986; **13**: 125–126.

Leader. Double blind or not? *British Medical Journal* 1970; **23**: 597–598.

Leary WE. Warning issued on 2 heart drugs after deaths of patients in a test. *New York Times* April 26, 1989.

Lehrer, T. *That Was the Year That Was*. New York: Reprise Records. No. 6179, 1965.

Leroux B, Rose J-P, Grun G *et al*. Traitement de la maladie des membranes hyalines par l'association plasminogè-urokinase. *La Nouvelle Presse Medicale* 1976; **5**: 699–702.

Levine RJ. *Ethics and Regulation of Clinical Research*. Baltimore: Urban & Schwartzenberg, 1981.

Levine C, Gallo G, Steinbock B. The case of Baby Jane Doe. *Hastings Center Report* 1984; **14**: 10–19.

Levenson T. *Measure for Measure.* New York: Simon and Schuster, 1994.

Lewis J. The humanitarian theory of punishment. *Res Judicatae* (Australia) 1952; **6**: 224–228.

Lidz CW, Meisel A. Informed consent and the structure of medical care. In: *Making Health Care Decisions: The Ethical and Legal Implications of Informed Consent in the Patient-Practitioner Relationship,* Volume 2. Washington: US Government Printing Office, 1983.

Lilienfeld AM, Pasamanick B. The association of maternal factors with the development of cerebral palsy and epilepsy. *American Journal of Obstetrics and Gynecology* 1955; **70**: 93–101.

Lock S. *A Difficult Balance: Editorial Peer Review in Medicine.* London: Nuffield Provincial Hospitals Trust, 1985.

Locke JC, Reese AB. Retrolental fibroplasia. The negative role of light, mydriatics, and the ophthalmoscopic examination in its etiology. *Archives of Ophthalmology* 1952; **48**: 44–47.

Louis TA, Bailar JC III, Lavori PW. Principles of clinical pharmacology. III. Experimental designs for clinical investigations. In: Lemberger L, Reidenberg (editors). *Proceedings of the Second World Conference on Clinical Pharmacology and Therapeutics.* New York: American Society for Pharmacology and Experimental Therapeutics, 1984.

Lomas J. Do practice guidelines guide practice? The effect of a consensus statement on the practice of physicians. *New England Journal of Medicine* 1989; **321**: 306–1310.

Ludmerer KM. *Genetics and American Society.* Baltimore: Johns Hopkins University Press, 1972.

Lynn J. Quoted in Hendin H. *Seduced by Death. Doctors, Patients and the Dutch Cure.* New York: WW Norton, 1997.

Lynn J, DeGrazia D. An outcomes model of medical decision-making. *Theoretical Medicine* 1991; **12**: 325–343.

Lyon J. *Playing God in the Nursery.* London: Norton, 1985.

Maas van der PJ. Changes in Dutch opinions on active euthanasia, 1966 through 1991. *Journal of the American Medical Association* 1995; **273**: 1411–1414.

MacDonald D. Cerebral palsy and intrapartum fetal monitoring. *New England Journal of Medicine* 1996; **334**: 659–660.

MacIntyre A. *Hume's Ethical Writings.* London: University of Notre Dame Press, 1965.

Mainland D. The use and misuse of statistics in medical publications. *Clinical Pharmacological Therapy* 1960; **1**: 411–422.

Mainland D. Statistical ritual in clinical journals: Is there a cure? *British Medical Journal* 1984; **288**: 920–922.

Manchester W. Manchester on leadership. *Modern Maturity* 1988; **January–February**: 8–11.

Mandel EM, Rockette HE, Bluestone CD *et al.* Efficacy of amoxicillin with and without decongestant-antihistamine for otitis media with effusion in children. *New England Journal of Medicine* 1987; **316**: 432–437.

Marquis D. Leaving therapy to chance. *Hastings Center Report* 1983; **13**: 40–47.

Marris P. *Loss and Change.* New York: Pantheon, 1974.

Mather HG, Pearson WG, Read KLQ *et al.* Acute myocardial infarction: home and hospital treatment. *British Medical Journal* 1971; **3**: 334–342.

Maynard A, Chalmers I. *Non-random Reflections on Health Services Research.* London: BMJ Publishing Group, 1997.

McCarthy M. US patients do not always get the best end-of-life care. *Lancet* 1997; **349**: 1747.

McNeill PM. *The Ethics and Politics of Human Experimentation.* Cambridge: Cambridge University Press, 1993.

Medawar PB. *Induction and Intuition in Scientific Thought. Jayne Lectures for 1968.* Philadelphia: American Philosophical Society, 1969.

Medawar PB. *The Limits of Science.* Oxford: Oxford University Press, 1984.

Medical Research Council. Streptomycin treatment of tuberculosis. *British Medical Journal* 1948; **ii**: 769–782.

Meittinen OS. *Theoretical Epidemiology. Principles of Occurrence Research in Medicine.* New York: John Wiley, 1985.

Meisel A, Roth LH. What we do and do not know about informed consent. *Journal of the American Medical Association* 1981; **246**: 2473–2477.

Miké V. Philosophers assess randomized clinical trials. The need for dialogue. *Controlled Clinical Trials* 1989; **10**: 244–253.

Miké V, Krauss AN, Ross GS. Symposium on ethics and clinical trials. Neonatal extracorporeal membrane oxygenation (ECMO): clinical trials and the ethics of evidence. *Journal of Medical Ethics* 1993; **19**: 212–218.

Miller BL. Autonomy and the refusal of lifesaving treatment. *Hastings Center Report* 1981; **11**: 22–28.

Miller J. Going unconscious. In: Silvers RB (editor). *Hidden Histories of Science.* New York: New York Review Books, 1995.

Milne R, Sackett D. Commentary: The message is in the medium. *British Medical Journal* 1995: 311: 1059–1060.

Moore DS. *Statistics. Concepts and Controversies.* San Francisco: W.H. Freeman, 1979.

Moore TJ. *Deadly Medicine. Why Tens of Thousands of Heart Patients Died in America's Worst Drug Disaster.* New York: Simon & Schuster, 1995.

Mortimer J. *Murderers and Other Friends.* New York: Viking, 1994.

Moscowitz EH, Nelson JL. The best laid plans. Special Supplement. *Hastings Center Report* 1995; **November–December**: S3–S6.

Moses LE. The series of consecutive cases as a device for assessing outcomes of intervention. *New England Journal of Medicine* 1984; **311**: 705–710.

Mother (A). Baby Doe (letter). *The Nation* February 25, 1984.

Moulton JB. Law and manners. *The Atlantic Monthly* 1924; **134**: 1–5.

Mulrow CD, Thacker SB, Pugh JA. A proposal for more informative abstracts of review articles. *Annals of Internal Medicine* 1988; **108**: 613–615.

Mumford L. *The Conduct of Life.* New York: Harcourt Brace, 1951.

Murray TH. The communities need more autonomy. *Hastings Center Report* 1994; **24**: 32–33.

Murton LJ, Doyle LW, Kitchen WH. Care of very low birthweight infants with limited neonatal intensive care resources. *Medical Journal of Australia* 1987; **146**: 78–81.

Nader L. Quoted in Jonsen A, Garland M. Critical issues in newborn intensive care. *Pediatrics* 1975; **55**: 756–768.

Navarro M. Into the unknown: AIDS patients test drugs. *New York Times* February 29, 1992.

Nelson JL. Taking families seriously. *Hastings Center Report* 1992; **22**: 6–12.

Neonatal Extracorporeal Life Support Registry. Ann Arbor, Michigan. University of Michigan, July 1990.

Nicholson RH (editor). *Medical Research with Children. Ethics, Law and Practice.* Oxford: Oxford University Press, 1986.

Nickel JC. Quoted in *New York Times* 16 April 1997.

Nuland SB. *How We Die.* New York: Knopf, 1994.

Office of Scientific Integrity Inquiry. *Report Covering Clinical Trials for Otitis Media Conducted at the Children's Hospital of Pittsburgh, 1990.* Washington DC, 1990.

O'Rourke PP, Crone RK, Vacanti JP *et al.* Extracorporeal membrane oxygenation and conventional medical therapy in neonates with persistent pulmonary hypertension of the newborn: A prospective randomized study. *Pediatrics* 1989; **84**: 957–963.

Ortega M, Ramos AD, Platzker AC *et al.* Early prediction of ultimate outcome in newborn infants with severe respiratory failure. *Journal of Pediatrics* 1988; **113**: 744–747.

Ounsted M. Causes, continua and other concepts. I. The 'continuum of reproductive casualty.' *Paediatric and Perinatal Epidemiology* 1987; **1**: 4–7.

Ounsted M, Moar VA, Cockburn J *et al.* Factors associated with the intellectual ability of children born to women with high risk pregnancies. *British Medical Journal* 1984; **288**: 1038–1041.

Owens WC, Owens EU. Retrolental fibroplasia in premature infants: II Studies on the prophylaxis of the disease. The use of alpha tocopheryl[sic] acetate. *American Journal of Ophthalmology* 1949; **32**: 1631–1637.

Palmer EA. Editorial. The continuing threat of retinopathy of prematurity. *American Journal of Ophthalmology* 1996; **122**: 420–423.

Palmer EA, Flynn JT, Phelps DL et al. Incidence and early course of retinopathy of prematurity. *Ophthalmology* 1991; **98**: 1628–1640.

Paneth NS *et al.* Strategies for the care of the very low birthweight infant. (In progress.)

Paris JJ, Crone RK, Reardon F. Physicians' refusal of requested treatment—the case of Baby L. *New England Journal of Medicine* 1990; **322**: 1012–1015.

Parsons T. *The Social System.* Glencoe: Free Press, 1951.

Partridge JC, Wall SN. Analgesia for dying infants whose life support is withdrawn or withheld. *Pediatrics* 1997; **99**: 76–79.

Paterson K, Bailar JC III. A review of journal peer review. In: Warren KS (editor). *Selectivity in Information Systems. Survival of the Fittest.* New York: Praeger, 1985.

Pauly PJ. *Controlling Life. Jacques Loeb and the Engineering Ideal in Biology.* Oxford: Oxford University Press, 1987.

Pauli W. Quoted in Segal LE. The unscientific charm of the big bang (letter). *New York Times* May 4, 1990.

Paulos JA. *Beyond Numeracy.* New York: Vintage Books, 1992.

Percival T. *Medical Ethics.* London: Russell, 1803.

Perlman JM. Intrapartum hypoxic-ischemic cerebral injury and subsequent cerebral palsy. *Pediatrics* 1997; **99**: 851–859.

Pernick MS. *A Calculus of Suffering*: Pain, Professionalism, and Anaesthesia in Nineteenth-Century America. New York: Columbia University Press, 1985.

Pernick MS. *The Black Stork.* New York: Oxford University Press, 1996.

Matthews WB, Jr, Budget officer of the National Institute of Neurological and Communicative Disorders and Stroke, June 1979, personal communication.

Peters DP, Ceci SJ. Peer review practices of psychological journals: fate of published journals submitted again. *Behavioral Brain Science* 1982; **5**: 187–255.

Peto R, Collins R, Gray R. Large-scale randomised evidence: large simple trials and overview of trials. *Annals of the New York Academy of Science* 1993; **703**: 314– 340.

Phoon CK. Parents often urge overtreatment (letter). *Pediatrics* 1993; **92**: 187–188.

Pinto-Martin JA, Riola S, Cuann A *et al.* Cranial ultrasound prediction of disabling and non-disabling cerebral palsy at age two in a low birth-weight population. *Pediatrics* 1995; **95**: 249–254.

Pless JE. The story of Baby Doe. *New England Journal of Medicine* 1983; **309**: 664–666.

Pocock SJ. *Clinical Trials.* Chichester: John Wiley & Sons, 1983.

Policy Research Incorporated. *Medical Practice Demonstration Project.* Baltimore, Maryland, 1979.

Popper KR. *Conjectures and Refutations. The Growth of Scientific Knowledge.* London: Routledge & Kegan Paul, 1962.

Porter R. Offering resistance. *New York Times* June 29, 1997.

Postman N. *Technopoly. The Surrender of Culture to Technology.* New York: Alfred A. Knopf, 1992.

Prescott RJ. Maximal acid output and risk of ulcer (letter). *Lancet* 1977; **i**: 595–596.

Price de S DJ. *Little Science, Big Science.* New York: Columbia University Press, 1963.

Price de S DJ. The development and structure of the biomedical literature. In: Warren KS (editor). *Coping with the Biomedical Literature.* New York: Praeger, 1981.

Proust M. *Remembrance of Things Past.* Volume 1. *Within a Budding Grove.* New York: Random House, 1932.

Quinn MW, Wild J, Dean HG *et al.* Randomised double-blind controlled trial of effect of morphine on catecholamine concentrations in ventilated preterm babies. *Lancet* 1993; **342**: 324–327.

Quinn S. Childhood's end. *Washington Post* November 15, 1994.

Rabi II. quoted in Gingerich O (editor). *The Nature of Scientific Discovery.* Washington: Smithsonian Institution Press, 1975.

Ramsey P. *The Patient as a Person: Explorations in Medical Ethics.* New Haven: Yale University Press, 1970.

Raphael DD. Moral sense. In: Weiner PE (editor). *Dictionary of the History of Ideas.* Volume III. New York: Charles Scribner's Sons, 1973.

Rawls J. *Political Liberalism.* New York: Columbia University Press, 1993.

Rennie D. Guarding the guardians: a conference on editorial peer review. *Journal of the American Medical Association* 1986; **256**: 2391–2392.

Rennie D. Editorial. The Cantekin Affair. *Journal of the American Medical Association* 1991; **266**: 3333–3337.

Rennie D, Flanagin A. The Second International Congress on Peer Review. *Journal of the American Medical Association* 1994; **272**: 91.

Renzong, Q. Economics and medical decision-making. *Seminars in Perinatology.* 1987; **9**: 262–263.

Report. *Medical Care of the Newborn in England and Wales.* London: Royal College of Physicians, 1988.

Report by the Committee on Government Operations. *Are Scientific Misconduct and Conflicts of Interest Hazardous to Our Health?* Washington DC: Government Printing Office, June 13, 1989.

Rest JR. *Development in Judging Moral Issues.* Minneapolis: University of Minnesota Press, 1979.

Rhoden N. Treating Baby Doe: The ethics of uncertainty. *Hasting Center Report* 1986; **16**: 34–42.

Robertson CMT, Hrynchyshyn GJ, Etches PC *et al.* Population-based study of the incidence, complexity, and severity of neurologic disability among survivors weighing 500 through 1250 grams at birth: A comparison of two birth controls. *Pediatrics* 1992; **90**: 750–755.

Roethlisberger FJ, Dickson WJ. *Management and Worker.* Cambridge, Massachusetts: Harvard University Press, 1939.

Rosenthal R, Jacobson L. *Pygmalion in the Classroom: Teacher Expectation and Pupil's Intellectual Development.* New York: Holt, Rinehart & Winston, 1968.

Roszak T. *The Cult of Information: The Folklore of Computers and the True Art of Thinking.* New York: Pantheon, 1991.

Rothman DJ. Introduction. In: Gaylin W, Glasser I, Marcus S, Rothman DJ (editors). *Doing Good. The Limits of Benevolence.* New York: Pantheon Books, 1978.

Rutstein DD. Should research design and scientific merits be evaluated? *Daedalus* 1969; **524**: 527–528.

Sackett DL. Bias in analytic research. *Journal of Chronic Disease* 1979; **32**: 51–63.

Sackett DL, Haynes RB, Tugwell P. How to read a clinical journal. In: *Clinical Epidemiology: A Basic Science for Clinical Medicine.* pp. 285–321. Boston: Little Brown, 1985a.

Sackett DL, Haynes RB, Tugwell P. *Clinical Epidemiology: A Basic Science for Clinical Medicine.* Boston: Little Brown, 1985b.

Saigal S, Furlong WJ, Rosenbaum PL *et al.* Do teens differ from parents in rating health- quality of life? A study of premature and control teen/parent dyads. *Pediatric Research* 1995a; **37**: 271A, Abstract No. 1610

Saigal S, Furlong WJ, Feeny DH *et al.* Parents' perceptions of the health-related quality of life of teenage extremely low birthweight and control children. *Pediatric Research*, Abstract No. 225, 1995b; **37**: 40A, Abstract No. 225.

Saigal S, Feeny DH, Furlong WJ et al. How premature teens perceive their own health- related quality of life: Comparison with controls. *Journal of the American Medical Association* 1996; **276**: 453–459.

Sameroff AJ, Chandler MJ. Reproductive risk and the continuum of caretaking casualty. *Review of Child Development Research* 1975; **4**: 187–244.

Sandham JD, Hull RD, Brant RF. Commentary. Pulmonary artery flow directed catheter: the evidence. *Lancet* 1996; **348**: 1324.

Sass HM. A critique of the Enquette Commission's report on gene technology. *Bioethics* 1988; **3**: 264–275.

Saugstad OD. Neonatal oxygen radical disease. In: David TJ (editor). *Recent Advances in Paediatrics.* Edinburgh: Churchill Livingstone, 1992.

Saunders RA, Donahue ML, Christman LM *et al.* Racial variation in retinopathy of prematurity. *Archives of Ophthalmology* 1997; **115**: 604–608.

Schechter NL, Blankson V, Pachter LM. The ouchless place: no pain, children's gain. *Pediatrics* 1997; **99**: 890–893.

Scheiber GJ, Poulier J-P. International health spending and utilization trends. *Health Affairs* 1988; **Fall**: 106.

Schilpp PA (editor). *The Philosophy of Karl Popper.* LaSalle, Illinois: Open Court, 1974.

Schneiderman LJ, Kaplan RM, Pearlman RA *et al.* Do physicians' own preferences for life-sustaining treatment influence their perceptions of patients' preferences? *Journal of Clinical Ethics* 1993; **4**: 28–32.

Schneiderman MA. The proper size of a clinical trial: Grandma's strudel method. *Journal of New Drugs* 1964; **January-February**: 3–11.

Schulz KF, Chalmers I, Hayes RJ *et al.* Empirical evidence of bias: dimensions of methodological quality associated with estimates of treatment effects in controlled trials. *Journal of the American Medical Association* 1995; **273**: 408–412.

Scott JES. Ethics in neonatal surgery. *Theoretical Surgery* 1987; **2**: 34–39.

Segelov E, Tattersall MHN, Coates AS. Redressing the balance—The ethics of *not* entering an eligible patient on a randomised trial. *Annals of Oncology* 1992; **3**: 103–105.

Seiberth V, Linderkamp O, Knorz MC. A controlled trial of light and retinopathy of prematurity. *American Journal of Ophthalmology* 1994; **118**: 492–495.

Seller MJ. The human embryo: a scientist's point of view. *Bioethics* 1993; **7**: 135–140.

Shapiro AK. A contribution to a history of the placebo effect. *Behavioral Science* 1960; **5**: 109–135.

Shaw GB. Preface on doctors. In: Shaw GB (editor). *The Doctor's Dilemma,* 1911.

Shaw LW, Chalmers TC. Ethics in cooperative clinical trials. *Annals of the New York Academy of Sciences* 1970; **169**: 487–495.

Shenai JP, Kennedy KA, Chytil F *et al.* Clinical trial of vitamin A supplementation in infants susceptible to bronchopulmonary dysplasia. *Journal of Pediatrics* 1987; **111**: 269–277.

Shenk D. *Data Smog.* San Francisco: Harper Edge, 1997.

Shepard G. A cradle in the twilight zone. *Express* 1990; **12** (March 30): 1–23.

Shipley JT. *Dictionary of Word Origins.* Totowa: Littlefield, Adams & Company, 1979.

Shorter E. *The Making of the Modern Family.* New York: Basic Books, 1975.

Shorter E. *From Paralysis to Fatigue. A History of Pyschosomatic Illness in the Modern Era.* New York: Free Press, 1992.

Sigerist HE. *Medicine and Human Welfare.* New Haven: Yale University Press, 1941.

Silverman WA. *Retrolental Fibroplasia. A Modern Parable.* New York: Grune & Stratton, 1980.

Silverman WA. Informed consent in customary practice and in clinical trials. In: Goldworth A, Silverman WA, Stevenson DK *et al.* (editors). *Ethics and Perinatology.* Oxford: Oxford University Press, 1995.

Silverman WA. Patients' preferences and randomised trials. *Lancet* 1996; **347**: 171–174.

Silverman WA. Equitable distribution of the risks and benefits associated with medical innovations. In: Maynard A, Chalmers I (editors). *Non-random Reflections on Health Services Research.* London: BMJ Publishing Group, 1997.

Silverman WA, Andersen DH, Blanc WA *et al.* A difference in mortality rate and incidence of kernicterus among premature infants alloted to two prophylactic regimens. *Pediatrics* 1956; **18**: 614–625.

Simes RJ, Tattersal MHN, Coates AS *et al.* Randomised comparison of procedures for obtaining informed consent in clinical trials for treatment of cancer. *British Medical Journal* 1986; **293**: 1065–1068.

Simon HA. *Administrative Behavior: A study of Decision-Making Processes in Administrative Organizations*, 3rd Edition. New York: Free Press, 1976.

Simons M. Dutch doctors to tighten rules on mercy killings. *New York Times* September 11, 1995.

Singer DE. Problems with stopping rules in trials of risky therapies: The case of warfarin to prevent stroke in atrial fibrillation. *Clinical Research* 1993; **41**: 482–486.

Singer P. A report from Australia: which babies are too expensive to treat? *Bioethics* 1987; **1**: 275–283.

Singer P. *Rethinking Life and Death.* New York: St. Martin's Press, 1994.

Singer P, Wells D. *The Reproduction Revolution.* Oxford: Oxford University Press, 1984.

Skolnick AA. Apgar quartet plays perinatologist's instruments. *Journal of the American Medical Association* 1996; **276**: 1939–1940.

Skrabanek P, McCormick J. *Follies and Fallacies in Medicine.* Glasgow: The Tarragon Press, 1989.

Smith R, Rennie D. And now, evidence based editing. *British Medical Journal* 1995; **311**: 826.

Smithells RW. Iatrogenic hazards and their effects. *Postgraduate Medicine* 1975; **15**: 39–52.

Snow CE. A discussion of the relation of illumination intensity to productive efficiency. *The Technical Engineering News* 1927; **2**: 9–14.

Society for Pediatric Epidemiologic Research (abstracts). Fourth Annual Meeting. *Paediatric and Perinatal Epidemiology* 1991; **5**: A1–A23.

Socrates. Quoted in Kass LR. *Toward a More Natural Science. Biology and Human Affairs.* New York: Free Press, 1991.

Soll RF. Neonatal extracorporeal membrane oxygenation—a bridging technique. *Lancet* 1996; **348**: 70–71.

Stahlman MI. Medical complications in premature infants. Is treatment enough? *New England Journal of Medicine* 1989; **320**: 1551–1553.

Standards [The] of Reporting Trials Group. A proposal for structured reporting of randomized controlled trials. *Journal of the American Medical Association* 1994; **272**: 1926–1931.

Sternberg M. *Josef Skoda (1815–1881).* Vienna: Springer, 1924.

Stevenson DK, Ariagno RL, Kutner JS *et al.* The 'Baby Doe' rule. *Journal of the American Medical Association* 1986; **255**: 1909–1912.

Stewart (Surgeon-General) WH. Clinical Investigations Using Human Subjects. Circulated (unpublished) memorandum dated February 8, 1966.

Stinson R, Stinson P. *The Long Dying of Baby Andrew.* Boston: Little Brown, 1983.

Streptomycin in Tuberculosis Trials Committee. Streptomycin treatment of pulmonary tuberculosis. *British Medical Journal* 1948; **i**: 769–782.

Sullivan JL. Iron metabolism and oxygen radical injury in premature infants. In: Lauffer RB (editor). *Iron and Human Disease.* Boca Raton, Florida: CRC Press, 1992.

Sullivan JL, Newton RB. Serum antioxidant activity in neonates. *Archives of Disease in Childhood* 1988; **63**: 748–750.

SUPPORT (the) Principal Investigators. A controlled trial to improve care for seriously ill hospitalized patients. *Journal of the American Medical Association* 1995; **274**: 1591–1593.

Taddio A, Stevens B, Craig K *et al.* Efficacy and safety of lidociaine-prilocaine cream for pain during circumcision. *New England Journal of Medicine* 1997; **336**: 1197–1201.

Terry TL. Extreme prematurity and fibroplastic overgrowth of persistent vascular sheath behind each crystalline lens. I. Preliminary report. *American Journal of Ophthalmology* 1942; **25**: 203–204.

Thomas L. *The Youngest Science.* New York: Viking, 1983.

Thomas L. What doctors don't know. *New York Review of Books* September 24, 1987.

Thoreau HD. *Walden.* New York: WW Norton, 1966 (first published in 1854).

Thucydides. *History of the Peloponnesian War (424 BC).* Quoted in Poundstone W. *The Prisoner's Dilemma.* New York: Anchor Books, 1993.

Till JE, Sutherland HJ, Meslin EM. Is there a role for preference assessments in research on quality of life in oncology? *Quality of Life Research* 1992; **1**: 31–40.

Tin W, Wariyar U, Hey E. Changing prognosis for babies of less than 28 week's gestation in the north of England between 1983 and 1994. *British Journal of Medicine* 1997; **314**: 107–111.

Tocqueville, quoted in Postman N. *Conscientious Objections.* New York: Vintage Books, 1988.

Torrance GW, Thomas WH, Sackett DL. A utility maximization model for evaluation of health programs. *Health Services Research* 1972; **7**: 118–133.

Tredgold T. quoted in Florman SC. *The Civilized Engineer.* New York: St. Martin's Press, 1987.

Treuherz J. *Hard Times: Social Realism in Victorian Art.* London: Lund Humphries, 1987.

Trials of War Criminals Before the Nuremberg Military Tribunals Under Council Law, No. 10. Volume 2. Washington, DC: Government Printing Office, 1949.

Tukey JW. The future of data analysis. *Annals of Mathematical Statistics* 1962; **33**: 1–67.

Tukey JW. Some thoughts on clinical trials, especially problems of multiplicity. *Science* 1977; **198**: 679–684.

Tversky A, Kahneman D. The framing of decisions and the psychology of choice. *Science* 1981; **211**: 453–458.

UK Collaborative ECMO Trial Group. UK collaborative randomised trial of neonatal extracorporeal membrane oxygenation. *Lancet* 1996; **348**: 75–82.

US Child Abuse Protection and Treatment Amendments of 1984. *Public Law 98–457.*

US Congressional Office of Technology Assessment. Cited in Freudenheim M. In pursuit of the punctual baby. *New York Times* December 28, 1988.

Veatch RM. Abandoning informed consent. *Hastings Center Report* 1995; **March-April**: 5–12.

Vere DW. Problems in controlled trials—a critical response. *Journal of Medical Ethics* 1983; **9**: 85–89.

Virgo JA. A statistical procedure for evaluating the importance of scientific papers. *Library Quarterly* 1977; **47**: 415–430.

Volgyesi FA. 'School for Patients' hypnosis therapy and psychoprophylaxis. *British Journal of Medical Hypnotism* 1954; **5**: 8–15.

Vollrath J. Experiments and rights. *Bioethics* 1989; **3**: 93–105.

Wachter RM. AIDS, activism, and the politics of health. *New England Journal of Medicine* 1992; **326**: 128–132.

Wachter de MAM. Euthanasia in the Netherlands. *Hastings Center Report* 1992; **March-April: 3–8.**

Walker CHM. '...officiously to keep alive.' *Archives of Disease in Childhood* 1988; **63**: 560–564.

Wallace I. The incredible Dr. Bell. In: Wallace I (editor). *The Sunday Gentleman.* New York: Simon and Schuster, 1965.

Walster JS, Cleary TA. A proposal for a new editorial policy in the social sciences. *American Statistician* 1970; **28**: 16–19.

Walton Sir J, quoted in Medical News. *British Medical Journal* 1987; **295**: 1003.

Warren KS. Qualitative aspects of the biomedical literature. In: Warren KS (editor). *Coping with the Biomedical Literature.* New York: Praeger, 1981.

Watts JL. Chapter 26. Retinopathy of prematurity. In: Sinclair JC, Bracken M (editors). *Effective Care of the Newborn Infant.* Oxford: Oxford University Press, 1992.

Webster C. *The Great Instauration. Science, Medicine and Reform 1626–1660.* London: Duckworth, 1975.

Weiss DJ. An experiment in publication: advance publication review. *Applied Psychological Measurement* 1989; **13**: 1–7.

Wennberg JE. Outcomes research, cost containment, and the fear of health rationing. *New England Journal of Medicine* 1988; **b 323**: 1202–1204.

Wennberg JE. What is outcomes research? *Institute of Medicine. Medical Innovations at the Crossroads. Volume 1: Modern Methods of Clinical Investigation.* Washington, DC: National Academy Press, 1990.

Wennberg JE, Mulley AG Jr, Henley D *et al.* An assessment of prostatectomy for benign urinary tract obstruction: geographic variations and the evaluation of medical care outcomes. *Journal of the American Medical Association* 1988; **a 259**: 3027–3030.

Werner ME, Bierman JM, French FE. *The Children of Kauai.* Honolulu: University of Hawaii Press, 1971.

Whyte WF. *Men at Work.* Homewood, Illinois: Dorsey Press, 1961.

Wilder T. *The Skin of Our Teeth.* New York: Samuel French, 1942.

Wilford JN. NASA plans new series of cheaper space craft. *New York Times* December 19, 1995.

Wilkinson DJ. Anaesthesia and surgery in children. *Lancet* 1987; **i**: 750.

Williams A. Beyond effectiveness and efficiency...lies equality. In: Maynard A, Chalmers I. (editors). *Non-random Reflections on Health Care Research.* London: BMJ Publishing Group, 1997.

Wolf AR. Treat babies, not their stress responses. *Lancet* 1993; **342**: 319.

Wolf S. Placebos: Problems and pitfalls. *Clinical Pharmacology and Therapeutics* 1962; **3**: 254–257.

Wolpert L. *The Unnatural Nature of Science.* Cambridge, Massachusetts: Harvard University Press, 1993.

Working Group on Recommendations for Reporting Clinical Trials in the Biomedical Literature. Call for comments on a proposal to improve reporting of clinical trials in the biomedical literature. *Annals of Internal Medicine* 1994; **121**: 894–895.

World Medical Association. *Declaration of Helsinki: Recommendations Guiding Medical Doctors in Biomedical Research.* Adopted by the 18th World Medical Assembly, Helsinki, Finland, 1964.

World Medical Association. *Declaration of Helsinki: Recommendations Guiding Medical Doctors in Biomedical Research.* Revised by the 29th World Medical Assembly, Tokyo, Japan, 1975.

World Medical Association. Declaration of Helsinki: Recommendations guiding physicians in biomedical research involving human subjects. *Journal of the American Medical Association* 1997; **277**: 925–926.

Worster D. *Under Western Skies: Nature and History in the American West.* New York: Oxford University Press, 1992.

Zenzes MT, Caspar RF. Cytogenics of human oocytes, zygotes and embryos after *in vitro* fertilization. *Human Genetics* 1992; **88**: 367–375.

Zupancic JAF, Gillie P, Steiner DL *et al.* Determinants of parental authorization for involvement of newborn infants in clinical trials (abstract). *Pediatrics* 1997; **99**: 116.

Index